Coming from a medical background Carrie, originally an RGN, retrained to her current position as Specialist in Musculoskeletal problems and has run her own clinic for over 25 years. During this time, she travelled overseas to research into the cause of bad backs since this was what most of her patients complained of. They encouraged her to write this book. It is her lifelong dream to leave a legacy that her book is used in schools to educate children on the correct way of doing activities of daily living that will prevent the aches and pains their peers now endure.

I dedicate this book to all the children of the world – may they use its contents to change their quality of life in their later years and be wise enough to pass the information onto their children.

Carrie Ransom

BREAK YOUR BAD HABITS

Before Your Aches and Pains Break You

AUSTIN MACAULEY PUBLISHERS™
LONDON · CAMBRIDGE · NEW YORK · SHARJAH

Copyright © Carrie Ransom 2023

The right of Carrie Ransom to be identified as author of this work has been asserted by the author in accordance with sections 77 and 78 of the Copyright, Designs and Patents Act 1988.

All rights reserved. No part of this publication may be reproduced, stored in a retrieval system, or transmitted in any form or by any means, electronic, mechanical, photocopying, recording, or otherwise, without the prior permission of the publishers.

Any person who commits any unauthorised act in relation to this publication may be liable to criminal prosecution and civil claims for damages.

A CIP catalogue record for this title is available from the British Library.

ISBN 9781398434967 (Paperback)
ISBN 9781398434974 (ePub e-book)

www.austinmacauley.com

First Published 2023
Austin Macauley Publishers Ltd®
1 Canada Square
Canary Wharf
London
E14 5AA

With grateful thanks to my patients for encouraging me to write this book.

Table of Contents

Introduction 11

Observational Research 13

Comparison Chart 14

Research Conclusion 16

Chapter 1 The Spine 17

Chapter 2 Look at Your Posture –Others Do!............ 23

Chapter 3 What Constitutes a Habit? 27

Chapter 4 Why Does the Body Compensate? 30

Chapter 5 The Importance of Pelvic Neutral............. 34

Chapter 6 Bad Habits 41

The Habits.. 45

Chapter 7 How to Change Your Habits and Carrie's 'Rule of Ninety' 110

How To Change a Habit... 112

Chapter 8 Other Factors Affecting Posture 119

Final Thoughts.. 123

Bibliography 124

Introduction

Welcome to a common-sense approach to posture, the bad habits we develop over time and how these bad habits create problems that can eventually lead to ailments such as back pain, hip and knee replacements, arthritis, neck pain, migraine and much more… Not to mention unsightly deformities of the body such as dowagers hump, round shoulders… Let me start by saying I do not consider myself to be an expert in this subject, but I do have over 26 years of experience in this field. My background is in NHS nursing. It was here that I was taught to lift and handle patients using *the latest* techniques and the *latest* pieces of equipment. However, the techniques and equipment were constantly changing depending on the 'flavour of the moment policy' adopted by the governing authority, so you were unsure what was correct, or worse still what effect it might have on you and your body. I retrained to my present position as a Musculoskeletal Injuries Specialist, where it quickly became apparent that the majority of the problems and pain people were presenting with in my clinic, stemmed mainly from repetitive bad habits adopted and/or learned from peers. Habits they seemed unaware of were wrong and that would eventually lead to future problems and pain. The content of this book intends to highlight those bad habits we have all developed and are using in everyday life! It will show you how to determine what your posture is at present, then identify the majority of bad habits we all seem to repeat as well as teach to others. It is important to remember to *apply* the new actions (habits) to similar ones, for example, the action (habit) of 'bending over' using our backs, to garden, is the same action (habit) as bending your back to tie shoelaces, you get the idea? It is vital to use this book to find the new habit that will correct both actions.

This book will not only be good for your body, in particular your spine, but also improve the quality of your life, as well as your breathing and your looks. Can't be bad, eh?

My Very Best Wishes,
Carrie

Observational Research

The contents of this book are based on common sense, derived from years of clinical practice and my observational research in a variety of countries. It was during my research between Western and Eastern countries, that I realised the cultural habits of the east were very different from that of the west! I could write another book on just these but to keep it simple, I have done a comparison chart on the next page that will explain my reasons behind this book. It shows that the western world overindulges in too many snack/junk/fast foods containing refined carbohydrates that our bodies find hard to process, so store as excess fat, causing us to feel bloated and sluggish. They also drain our energy, leading us to take in too little exercise, coupled with excess gadgets to make life 'easier' leading to excessive weight gain (Sissan's article 2020). The Asians eat very little processed foods, dairy, or carbohydrates, though sadly the western influence and fast foods are slowly creeping in! Their diet at present consists mainly of fresh meat, fish, vegetables and fruit.

Comparison Chart

Habit	Western	Asian
Bending over	Upper body bends forward using the lower back as a hinge	Knees are bent in squat position which keeps back straight
Diet	Mainly carbohydrates, junk food and refined/processed foods	Mainly fresh veg, fruit, meat. Sticky rice is usually main source of Carbs (western foods are being introduced!)
Toilet habits	Sit down on a toilet	Squat over a hole in the ground
Exercise	Choice minority participation	Generational encouragement
Culture	Freedom of choice	Regimented
Lifestyle	Good quality for all	2-tier system but vast numbers of poor
Medical	UK: NHS Europe/USA: have very good healthcare system, mostly derived from insurance	The rich afford the best. The poor **have** to look after their own health. No insurance means they have to do their best to maintain it.

From the chart findings I was able to deduce that:

- Westerners bend from their upper bodies using their spines and not their thigh muscles which will atrophy through lack of use. This group of muscles is vital in providing strength for elevating as well as stabilising the body in most activities of daily living (see bad habits chapter).
- My observation revealed the majority of Asians were slender in stature. Therefore, there would be no excess loading on their joints.
- Because most Asian homes have a hole in the ground for their toilet, they needed to squat to perform. This means they *have* to use their 'quads' to push up their upper bodies. It may be one of the main reasons they stay slim as the larger you are the harder it is to push yourself up.
- The majority of Asians indulge in some sort of daily exercise. With no NHS system, the onus is solely on the individual to ensure they keep healthy since medical expenses are to most – prohibitive! Every morning thousands would flock to the parks to do some sort of exercise, either as an individual or as part of a group, the latter meant that their psychological needs were also taken care of since they socialised with others. Westerners tend to 'stay' in their own homes, don't/won't mix with others, making them feel isolated, introverted and depressed!
- Asian cultures still have old family traditions, looking after their families if old or ill. In the west, children have moved away from their birthplace. In addition, care homes are now a thriving industry.
- I did not see anyone in a wheelchair, electric buggy, or using a Zimmer/rollator frame, or any other aiding device since they didn't seem to require it.

Research Conclusion

I can only conclude that the reduction in carbohydrates (particularly the refined variety), meant that the majority of Asians were slim but strong. In addition, regular outdoor exercise not only strengthened and kept their bodies agile and supple but also kept their minds alert as well as fulfilled their social needs by interacting with other like-minded people. It was while I was in China that I spoke to a group of very slim old men with leathery skin who were all squatting, playing cards, through my interpreter, I was told the oldest was 91 and he came to the park daily because he enjoyed the company and a bit of gambling! I was in awe that these men had no trouble standing up unaided from this squatting position proving conclusively in my mind that the quadriceps thigh muscle is the key to why they didn't suffer the back problems we do in the west! Strengthen these and make small changes to our habits and we too can enjoy a better quality of life now and in our later years.

Chapter 1
The Spine

It is important that you understand a little of the workings of the spine in order that you might appreciate the need to protect it. We are first formed from a head and a tail, this is the sperm and the egg. The sperm fertilises the egg which becomes implanted in the womb. It starts to grow and again takes the form of a head and a tail (see pic below & next page).

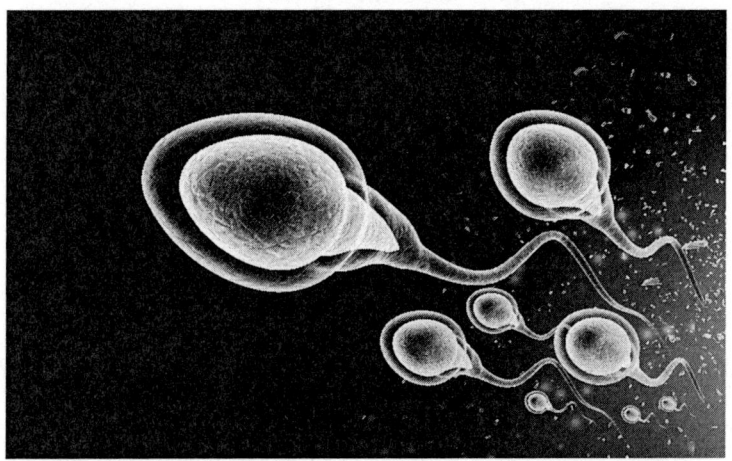

Sperm with head and tail

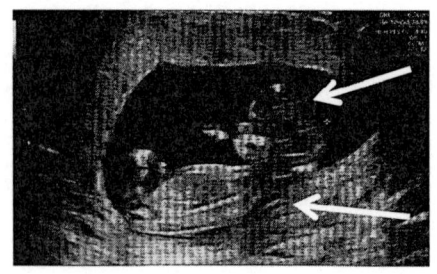 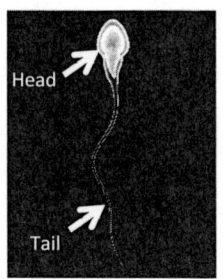

Foetus growing in the womb   Head and Spine

Let's look at what grows from the head: the ears, nose, mouth and eyes but the main growth is the most impressive complex computer in the world – our brain!

Now let us look at what grows from the tail: the neck, shoulders, arms, hands, torso with *all* the vital organs; heart, lungs, etc. As well as the pelvis, legs, feet and all the intricate digits of fingers and toes.

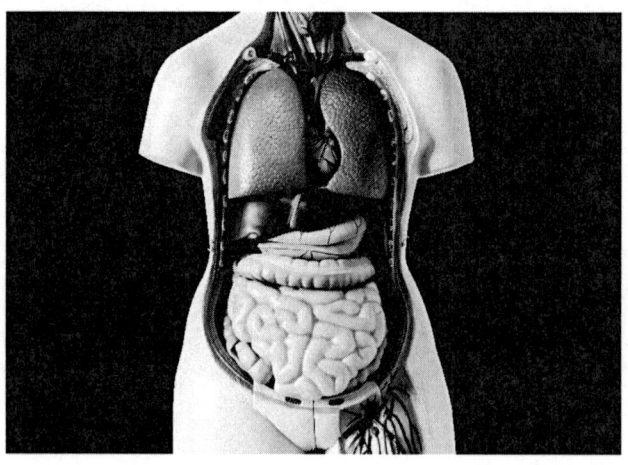

That tail is our **spine!**

Therefore, it is logical to assume that problems happening to the body, below the head (not originating from either direct or indirect trauma), h*ave* to emanate from the spine – wouldn't you agree? My years of professional experience and research have revealed it is the learned habits (the way we do an action) that you have seen and copied from your peers when you were younger that are the major contributory factor in damaging your spine that causes the pain to your body.

One of the most common offending examples of this can be seen in chapter 4, lifting incorrectly. We only get *one* spine so doesn't it makes sense to protect and look after it?

Put it like this, if we were given a top of the range car at birth and told this is your car but it is the Only car you will ever own… How well would you look after that car?

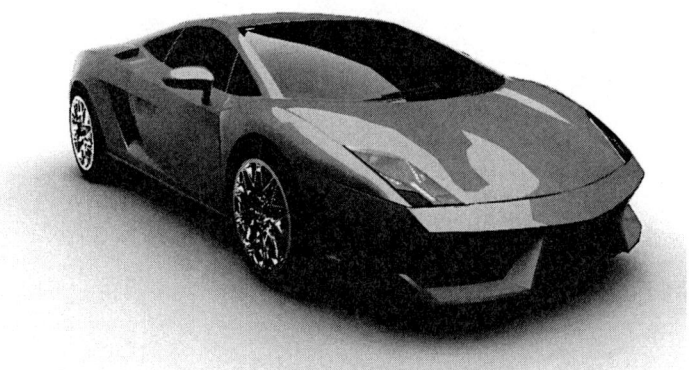

Bad habits taught and allowed to develop in early life will damage the spine as we grow causing untold problems for us later on.

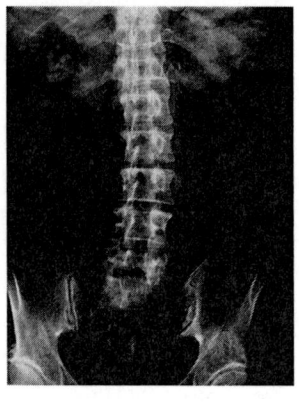

Damaged spine from repetitive bad habits

If the learned habits aren't changed and corrected, you will also create your own damaged spine. Worse still, you will pass on your habits to your children. Unless this cycle is broken, it will continue forever! How sad is that? We have to reverse this!

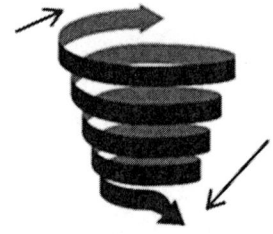

As we now know the spine represents all the body so you won't be surprised to know that patients have come to me with symptoms such as hip, knee and foot pain, bladder and bowel problems, migraine, carpal tunnel symptoms, fibromyalgia, indigestion, persistent coughs to name but a few! All were reversed when their misaligned spine was corrected, and unfortunately, the majority were caused by repetitive bad habits that put a strain on that particular part of the spine and finally a 'last straw' moment meant that the corresponding vertebra twisted out of alignment, irritating the nerve pathway causing their pain. That nerve pathway excites the muscles on a constant basis, they contract, creating the symptom(s) the patient presents with in the clinic. Once the vertebra(e) was corrected, strengthening exercises given and the New Habit(s) instilled, the problem went… Permanently!

I hope by now you can see the importance of protecting the spine and realise that most of the problems you have, have unfortunately been caused by the actions *you* do on a *daily* basis!

Review of the chapter

- We are formed from a head and tail.
  The *head* expands to permit the growth of the brain while the *tail* grows into the spine from which everything else grows.
- We know if there is no direct trauma to our body the likelihood of our source of pain will be coming from the spine.
- We now realise the importance of the spine and must protect it!
- We accept actions we currently do, harm the spine and so need changing.
- We must learn these new habits and teach them to our friends and relatives

Chapter 2
Look at Your Posture –Others Do!

Look at your posture...

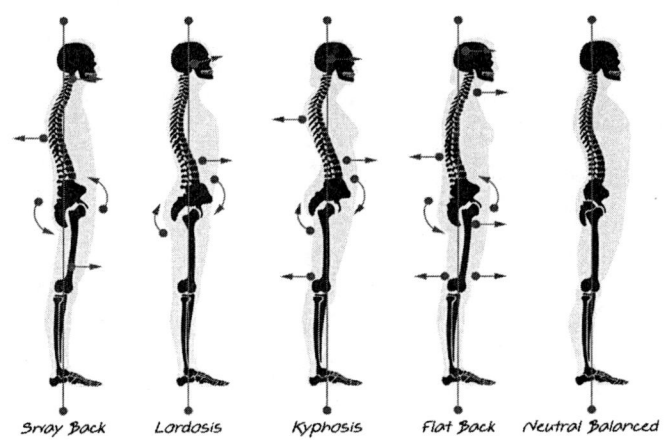

Sway Back   Lordosis   Kyphosis   Flat Back   Neutral Balanced

...others do

It is a fact that when we look in a mirror, we very rarely look at our posture, more what we are wearing rather than how we are wearing it? In the picture above we can see a variety of different postural positions. To identify yours, you may need the help of a friend but if you are on your own then just stand sideways in front of a mirror in undergarments then turn your head toward the mirror and observe where; your head is, your shoulders are, your bottom is, and which way your feet are pointing e.g. are they facing straight forward, are your toes pointing inwards or at an angle of ten to two?

It is important to know what postural shape you are in because this will help you to determine what areas of the body are being strained and will need help correcting these in order to prevent problems later in your life (some have already been mentioned).

Clearly, it would be of great benefit to our bodies if we were to have good posture, where muscle and skeletal loading are well balanced. Let us take a look at the difference good posture and bad posture creates.

Good Posture

- Look more confident
- Clothes fit and look more stylish
- Healthier for the body – more oxygen to lungs and therefore to the brain
- Prevents pain, RSI and long-term problems
- Body appears thinner/taller

Bad Posture

- Looks awkward
- Clothes fit badly
- Oxygen deficit making you tired and confused
- Long term damage to the body
- Appear shorter/larger

When you stand with the correct posture you 'appear' to have an air of authority about you that says you are confident and know what you are about, even if inside you are shaking like jelly! And trust me I know what that feels like (picture on right).

Now take a look at the picture on the left and ask yourself, if you were an employer, which one of these would you employ if they walked into an interview like that…?

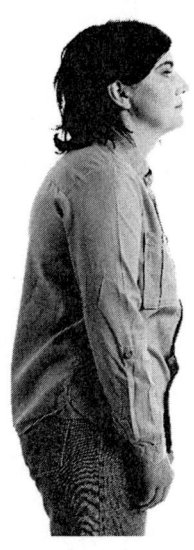 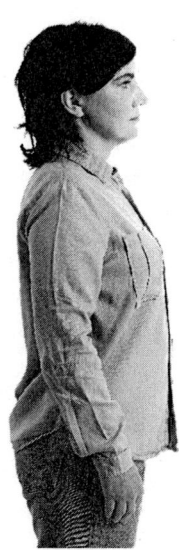

The clothes on the picture on the left look sagging and ill-fitting, and the posture gives off the 'am I bovvered?' attitude, (even if she is), whereas the picture on the right looks tailored and slender, and her posture indicates to us that she is confident, keen and has a professional attitude.

Regarding the 'healthier for body' postural good habit, I will not bore you with too much medical detail, but just so you know that at the bottom of the rib cage is a muscle called the diaphragm. This is vital for controlling the in/out breathing mechanism, therefore, if you hunch over or round your shoulders you will be squashing the diaphragm preventing the body from getting the full amount of air/oxygen into the body. This causes a chain reaction – lack of oxygen means the heart can't function as well, therefore it can't supply the rest of the body's cells with the vital oxygen, especially the brain and muscles; if the brain doesn't have enough oxygen several things happen: it fogs up your thinking, you feel tired and it becomes harder to make decisions or even function. If the muscles don't have enough oxygen, then all movement becomes an effort to do and any movement/action you do make will mean your muscles will tire much quicker.

By standing with the correct posture, you will appear to be taller and thinner not to mention that your body will not ache in the strained areas, e.g., low back, between the shoulder blades, this is because your muscular weight is now evenly distributed over your frame (skeleton). If you adopt this posture in standing, you can do it in walking and also in running so much less chance of sports injuries!

Chapter 3
What Constitutes a Habit?

A habit, whether good or bad is a movement or action that is done on a repetitive basis. It is an action that when done for the *first* time, produces *no* ill effects, repercussions or dire consequences such as pain. It is because there are no consequences that this action deceives the brain into thinking it is 'safe' to do. The brain subsequently allows the body to repeat this action until after some 1000 repetitions or when regularly performed, anywhere between 2–8 months, it becomes 'a habit'! (Research psychologist P Lally.) Regular repetition of the action allows the brain to store this information so we are able to perform this action **without** thinking about it, this is known as a Habit or an autonomous action! Consequently, if that habit is a bad one (see chapter 6), the person will be unaware that repetition of this action will create wear and tear on that part of the body and will cause problems and pain later in their life.

Good and bad habits are both formed and learned from a very early age and continue to be formed throughout our lives as we use our experience and reasoning to create new ones. At around six months old we spend most of our time looking around us soaking up what we see, keen to repeat the action and try it out as soon as we are able to. In addition, our guardians, parents and peers influence the way we do things since they are with us most of the time and teach us the way 'they have always done it' as well as the way 'they were taught' (though this book will show it will not necessarily have been the right way). As we continue through life we adapt the actions to suit ourselves and the required task, finding the quickest and easiest way to do that action. When we don't have consequences from that action, we assume all is well and continue doing it this way from then on. It is because we have adapted the way we do that action, that puts our bodies under strain, creating imbalances within the muscles, skeleton and spine. This is known as incorrect muscle loading. Repetition of a bad habit will cause an imbalance of the muscles making one side of our body weak while the other is overused (strained). Movement is created when muscles that are connected from one end of a bone to another (and this includes the spine) are stimulated by the brain's electrical impulses causing contraction (shortening) of those muscles that move the bone. Therefore, overused muscles will become strained and pull at their attachments. Take a look at the diagrams on the next page to see just how many muscles we have.

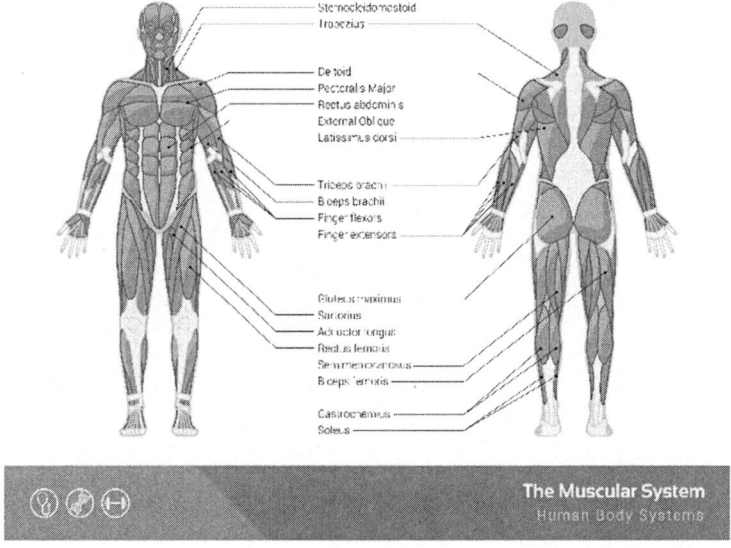

Note: most of the back ones are connected to the spine!

Review of the Chapter

- Habits are developed by what we see and do as a youngster, and then added to as we grow and learn to find a 'quicker and easier way' of doing everyday actions.
- 'Habits' are repetitious actions that incur no initial consequences so our brain allows us to repeat them.
- Habits form after 1,000 repetitions or when regularly done over a short period of time.
- Repetitive bad habits, manifest themselves later in life when they will cause problems, pain and discomfort.

Chapter 4
Why Does the Body Compensate?

The human body has the most intricate computer (brain) you are ever likely to come across. Thousands have tried to understand how the body works and still, it mystifies them. The normal body stands perpendicular to gravity (at right angles to the ground), the muscles of our bodies are arranged to promote this. Because muscles work in pairs when one contracts the other relaxes, most of you will know of the biceps and triceps muscles that move the upper arm. Therefore, if one or both pairs of muscles are weak it will put a strain on the attachments (bone ends) and as a consequence, it will have a direct effect on the body's posture, that is, the body will be pulled towards the stronger muscles, thus moving it away from perpendicular (correct/straight posture). Furthermore, when the body is injured or put under strain, it tries various methods to protect us from further injury, now without getting too technical, I will try to explain how it does this and why.

Firstly, I will need to tell you about the physics of lifting; the load, fulcrum and exertion; as an example, bending over to do an action, such as to pick up an object (the way most people do). The majority of people I have observed keep their knees either straight or only slightly bent, this uses their backs (mainly lower spine) when they lift. This action means that the whole of the top half of the body as well as what it is being lifted now becomes the load! This action will create wear and tear at this point. If done on a regular basis will cause the lower spine and its surrounding structures to become inflamed, initially producing aches and after a time, pain.

The spine's constant bending over can be likened to that of a metal bar being bent then straightened continuously, eventually, the stressed part (at the bend) will *snap!* Fortunately, we are not metal. However, the constant wear and tear on the lower spine is an accident waiting to happen, eventually creating a vertebral misalignment or even worse, a slipped disc! So imagine when there is a load to be picked up, this will add extra strain at the fulcrum (lower spine), so there is a huge risk of damage being done to the spine, especially if the action is repeated on a regular basis e.g., a brick layer, picking up a child, etc.

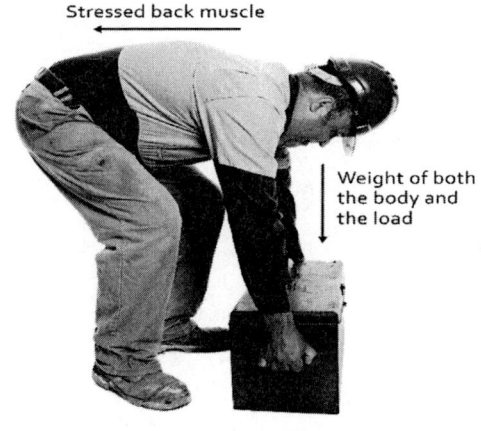

The picture on the previous page shows the action spoken about, highlighting where the wear and tear on the spine will occur when using the bad habit of bending the back to pick things up. Note: This is where most people have back pain!

If the body is continuously used in this way, the brain recognises that body part is *becoming* inflamed and will have already given out signals to the person, that is, it creates heat, aches and or pain in that area to let them know there is a problem. The response is usually rest and/or ice, and/or taking anti-inflammatory tablets. The latter will only serve to mask the problem for a while and if the action creating the problem stops, the pain usually goes away. If not, the body, no longer able to cope, will do one of two things: it will either attempt to put a protective layer around the inflamed area in order to restrict that movement in an effort to prevent the situation from becoming worse, or it will get the body to do the action in a different way so as not to create the pain… the latter is known as a compensatory movement. This compensatory movement means that the body will have moved away from the pain to allow you to continue doing that action and will now be using that set of particular muscles in a different way, creating an unequal loading i.e., one of the pairs of muscles will become weak and the other will be overused/strained. The whole process will now begin again in the new compensatory position and will eventually create problems at the new loading place, also causing problems for the compensatory muscles.

So as you can see unfortunately the body tends to compensate if it can't correct. But the worse part of this is that you won't even know it, your body will just do it on your behalf! This creates enormous problems for health professionals since they tend to treat the presenting problem (symptoms) and *not* the cause!

However, all of this can be avoided to a much less degree, by using the correct method to do an action in the first instance thus protecting the body in particular the back/lower spine.

Review of the Chapter

- When we injure or repetitively strain our body it forms layers around that area to protect it from further injury.
- Loading the body wrongly puts strain on the fulcrum (the lumbar Spine). If we were metal, we would snap!
- The body compensates automatically by finding a different way to achieve the objective.
- Compensations create other problems elsewhere making correct diagnosis of the cause, very difficult.

Chapter 5
The Importance of
Pelvic Neutral

In this chapter, I want to demonstrate how putting/keeping the pelvis in 'neutral' while doing an action can protect the lower spine. With the added bonus of making you look as if you have lost half a stone... instantly!!! ☺ In order to do that I need to explain the structure of the spine. The lower spine has a natural forward/anterior curve see picture below. Therefore, if there is loading or postural strain/stress in a forward direction i.e., if the action you are doing involves you bending your back in a forward motion, it will put pressure on the discs (between each vertebra) squeezing them.

This repeated action causes compression of the disc and weakens its corresponding vertebra. Any futuristic bend and twisting movement, may become the 'last straw' whereupon that vertebra will misalign! If this happens the disc is forced out to one side, becomes inflamed and will eventually press on its nerve causing pain anywhere along its nerve pathway (commonly know as a trapped nerve). For example, the lumbar spine supply the nerves of the lower body so pain can ensue anywhere from the abdomen to the feet/toes.

The pictures on the next page show the strain put on the lower spine when seated incorrectly in the different positions. The picture on the right shows an anterior tilted pelvis. The lower back is arched, the belly button pointing towards the floor, compressing the lumbar (lower) spine and its discs.

So many of us do this habit which is created by the bad habit of tucking our feet underneath the chair, and/or rocking our upper body forward so as to rest our elbows on a table, and definitely, if we wrap our feet around the front legs of the chair, this habit particularly applies to short people whose legs do not touch the ground. The middle picture shows sitting in the pelvic neutral position where the back is kept straight and the body's load is equally divided between front and back. The picture on the next page marked posterior tilt, is usually done by people who 'slouch' on chairs and couches (don't sit squarely on the chair). This forces the vertebrae of the lumbar spine inwards and creates another more serious problem for the disc.

In the same way standing in anterior tilted pelvis (bottom stuck out/tummy button pointing to the floor) will cause crushing of the lumbar discs, this can have a domino effect on the pelvic core stability, which can interfere with internal structures such as the womb, prostate, bladder etc. Posterior pelvic tilt where the belly button points upward towards the ceiling, will put strain on the lower as well as mid and upper spine since it opposes the natural curve of the spine. While standing in 'pelvic neutral', the spine is held straight and strong because the muscular loading on the spine is equalled both at the back and the front.

We can conclude that having your spine out of neutral causes compression on the spine at certain points. Therefore, standing or sitting regularly in anterior or posterior tilted pelvis will compress the discs of the lumbar spine squeezing out

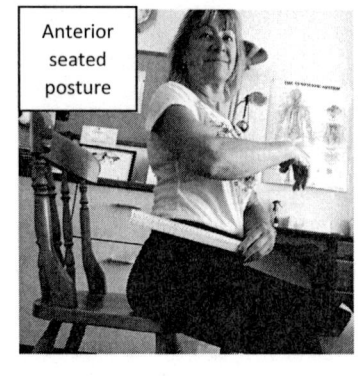

Anterior seated posture

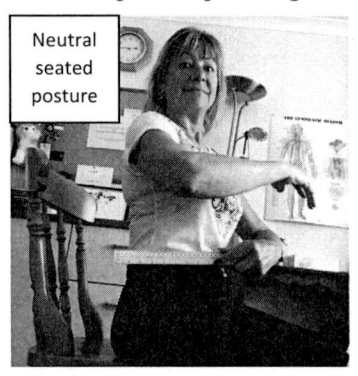

Neutral seated posture

vital fluid needed to maintain their shape so that they then can't perform their function as shock absorbers that keep the vertebral bones safe, preventing them from rubbing on each other (causing arthritis literal translation = bone inflammation).Years of bad postural habits will mean the discs will be unlikely to regain their natural shape/size, resulting in permanent damage to the back/spine narrowing the discs causing a condition known as, degenerative disc disease (DDD). If you were to add to this, any other bad habits you

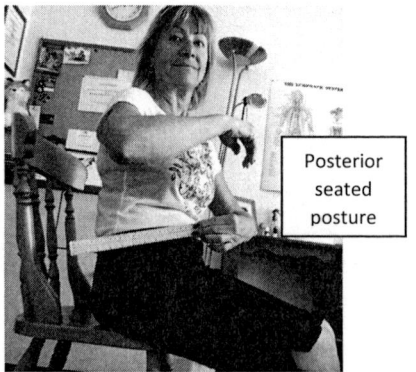

Posterior seated posture

may have, the time scale for that damage to occur is significantly reduced. In addition, it will be further reduced if your job and/or hobby involves bending with or without loads of heavy weights – it then becomes an accident waiting to happen!

It is vital for your body to avoid ALL of these things. You must *retrain your habit(s)* and learn to sit, stand and lift in *'pelvic neutral'*.

How to acquire 'Seated' pelvic neutral

Locate a hard wooden seat e.g., dining chair and sit squarely on it with your bottom well back in the seat and your back straight (at 90 degrees to your pelvis). Now with the back straight, rock the hip bone forward so it arches your lower back, you will now be in the forward-tilted position (see the picture of anterior tilted pelvis). Now let your bottom roll backward as if trying to push the base of the spine into the bottom of the chair back (see the picture of posterior tilted pelvis), repeat these actions rocking backward and forward, as you do so, become aware that your body rises and lowers as you transfer from front to back. You will also notice the (hard) bony lump in your bottom as you move back and forth. That bony lump is the pelvic bone, try to stop at the highest point i.e., directly on the bony prominence – **this is pelvic neutral!** You will need to practice this regularly so that this postural position becomes automatic when you sit.

Pelvic neutral when standing/walking

This is a little more difficult both to explain and to teach but teach it I will and learn it you must! That said, however, most men should be good at this since the movement of the pelvis is used automatically to obtain the pelvic thrust movement for penetration when making love.

How to acquire standing pelvic neutral

Stand naked sideways onto a full-length mirror. Observe your posture, locate your belly button and note if it points towards the floor or up towards the ceiling, there will only be a slight difference but it will be there, also note the type of posture you have (Chapter 2).

Now for the hard part, keeping your legs straight, knees locked do not move your upper body at all, make an arch with your back by pushing your tummy/abdomen out and forward allowing the pelvis to tip forward so you feel pressure in the lower back, this is the anterior tilt. Now in the same starting position try to flatten out your lumbar spine, it will help if you squeeze in the buttocks, you will be aware that your pelvis tips upwards (imagine you are standing in front of a shopping trolley and both your hands are full of shopping bags and you need to push the trolley forwards with your hips), this thrust action is what you will be using to achieve posterior pelvic tilt. It might be helpful to note that when you are in pelvic neutral you should feel your muscles tighten in your front upper thighs (quads) and in your lower front abdomen. It is in this position that when you look in the mirror you will look as if you have lost half a stone since it immediately flattens out your tummy bulge. Obtaining pelvic neutral takes time to achieve so don't worry, chances are you won't achieve this first time around, I didn't! Just keep practising it will come to you, I promise.

The Human Pendulum

Another helpful exercise is to stand up, feet forward and hip width apart. Whole body is soldier-like rigid. Now slowly rock your whole body forward, feeling your body weight transfer over your toes (don't let your heels come off the floor) now slowly let the body weight go back and over the heels (again don't let the toes come off the floor). Continue, slowly then if you can, close your eyes and be aware of where your body weight is then stop when you can feel your weight is even over the toes and heels.

Lifting in pelvic neutral

If you can learn to put your pelvis in neutral every time you lift you will be really protecting your lower spine. It just takes practice. With fully bent knees, and back straight, tilt the pelvis into anterior tilt now maintain this tilt throughout the lift of the object ensuring you use the front thighs to push your body upright, and keep the object as close to the body as possible. To set heavy weights down simply reverse the process; tilt the pelvis into anterior tilt and then bend the knees keeping the back *straight*, allow the upper body to go down with gravity. Once the object is placed on the floor, come up the same way as for lifting with a weight maintaining anterior tilt, this ensures you are using 'core' and not your spine. The more you use this action the faster it will become a good habit that will protect your lower back as well as strengthen those quads! This particularly applies when doing one-sided work e.g., pull-starting a petrol lawn mower, shovelling earth, etc.

Review of the Chapter

- Learning pelvic neutral in sitting and standing.
- Find postural neutral – the human pendulum
- Identifying anterior (forward) and posterior (back) tilt positions
- How to lift and set down in pelvic neutral

Chapter 6
Bad Habits

Before we start on this chapter, I want to try and impress upon you the two sayings I have which have helped me overcome my bad habits:

**It's not WHAT action you do…
It's HOW you do it.**

If how you do an action is 'quicker and easier'… it's usually *wrong*!!!

These sayings remind us *not* to take shortcuts when doing an action. My experience shows taking shortcuts will come back to bite us in the 'proverbial' in the long term! And it *is* the long term we are talking about since we all want to grow up without aches and pains and *not* have it enforced upon us that these are part of the ageing process because believe me when I tell you, they are *not!*

In chapter 3 we learned that to change a habit takes time and/or repetition. However, when we make our minds up to change a bad habit the new way of doing that action will feel strange, maybe even a little difficult at first. But, like any habit, it gets easier the more you rehearse it. Trust me, I speak from years of having to change most of these habits! Now they just come second nature and occasionally I stop and go to tell myself off, then realise that I actually did it the correct way. Lesson: when you do change from a bad to a good habit/action, make sure you give yourself praise, don't just chastise yourself when you do it wrong.

My tip: When you do an action, try to think of it as if it were doing a 'workout' because you know that it is doing your body good. That way you will be able to accept the 'different from normal' movement better and adopt the good habit sooner. You will actually be giving your body a workout since you will be using muscles that you haven't used for a long time because initially those muscles will be weak and ache but continued use will make them stronger.

My Tip: Get your eyes tested regularly. If you can't see properly, you will create your own bad habits. In my experience you will take your head closer to the item, not the other way around, this will lead to neck and upper back problems.

The list below has been drawn up as the most common bad habits performed by the majority of us on a daily basis. The list is by no means exhaustive. My advice would be to apply the principles to the action you are doing for example; the wrong action (bad habit) of bending your back with legs straight to tie your shoelaces, needs changing to the right action. Therefore, any action that involves 'bending the back' must be done in the correct way. The correct way to tie your shoelaces would be to go onto one knee, this keeps your back straight. Applying other bad habits would be things like gardening etc.

When you look at the list below you will realise that nearly all the actions you do will need tweaking in some way. Don't panic! This is quite normal. Most of the bad habits identified *were* mine!

My Tip: Do yourself a favour make a list of your bad habits. Put them in order of worst (most repetitive/harmful) and then pick the top three to correct. Once these are good habits i.e., they are now automatic, then take the next three and so on, until most of your bad habits have been changed.

NB. To try and correct all the bad habits at once will throw your brain into confusion and your psyche will have a meltdown so you will be destined to fail from the start.

Remember: be as quick to praise yourself as you are to chastise yourself.

My Tip: If your habit is something you do at work, then ask colleagues to point it out to you (they love being given permission for this). They will be doing you a huge favour.

Also, if you have children around give them permission to tell you off when you do the bad habit, they will be more than happy to oblige. Again, it will help you in the long run AND you will be teaching them the correct way of doing this action since they learn from you; a win-win situation!

Some readers may think they are too old to change their habits whilst some may take the changing too literal, possibly becoming overzealous, becoming rigid in the new position. Please know that as living beings our bodies are capable of many things including change – it is our minds we need to convince!!! Therefore, as suggested, take the three most important bad habits and practise getting into the new habit position hold it there for a few seconds then *relax* into this position. There is no need to be a 'soldier' apart from looking silly, you won't be able to sustain this rigid position for long and may revert back to your old habit!

The Habits

As mentioned, the list below is not exhaustive and is in no specific order, so go through them one at a time and pick out the ones you know you do, then repeat the task, this time asking someone if they have seen you do that habit. Believe me they will love to tell you!

1. Getting in/out of bed

The majority of us do this habit every day of our lives. You would think that you don't need to be advised the best way to get in/out of bed? However, my experience has shown otherwise.

Most of us just pull back the covers and 'jump' in. To get out, most pull back the covers and lift our head and upper bodies, we twist our legs over the side of the bed to put them on the floor and stand up. This action puts all the strain on the lower back added to all the other bad habits, may just be the 'last straw' with the possible consequence of a misalignment of the lower spine and the pain that goes with it (see chapter 8). This is because most of us do not have strong tummy muscles (abdominals) which means as you attempt to raise your upper body from the bed, your tummy will try to help but will fail miserably, as a consequence will then put all the strain on the back muscles and spine.

The Safe Way

It does not matter what side of the bed you sleep on… Turn over onto your side facing the edge of the bed, with knees bent and *keeping* your feet and ankles **tight** together as if they have been *tied* at the knees and ankles, place your hand that is facing the ceiling, palm down on the bed by your head, push up on this hand to raise your head and shoulders off the bed, so the under arm can now be positioned to support you by the elbow. Take the feet over the side of the bed and allow them to start to drop to the floor, this counterbalances the upper body that now wants to start rising off the bed, until it becomes upright, assist this by pushing up with the hand on the bed until you are sat in the upright position. For tummy strengthening exercises see chapter 8.

To get into bed

Just reverse this action, that is, sit on the side of the bed keep your feet and knees tight together, lean toward the pillow and as your upper body starts to go down, ease it with your elbow nearest the bed by placing this on the bed, as your upper body starts to go onto the bed your feet and knees will start to come up (counterbalancing your body) so you can just lift them a tad so they can rest on the bed. In this position simply roll onto your back. You are now in bed.

2. Turning over in bed (See the subconscious mind)

Most of us dig our heels into the foot of the bed then use our necks/shoulders to push the rest of our bodies under and through. This is both laboured and dangerous. Just consider the pressure you have just put on your neck! Especially if you have difficulty in turnover because of excess weight!!!

The Safe Way

Is similar to getting in/out of bed. If you are on your right side and you want to go onto your back or to your left, bend your knees keep them and ankles *tight* together and move them in the direction you want to go. Because they are tight together acting like a solid block they form the start of a human corkscrew for the rest of your body to follow the direction.

3. Lying on your front sunbathing/in bed

This is extremely hazardous for your spine since my experience tells me those that do this have a favourable side they always turn their head to which puts a huge strain on the neck vertebrae. If you sleep or lie for any length of time on your front, the neck muscles are over strained in one position, when the body needs to move to prevent pressure area damage (it has an inbuilt alarm telling us to move when lying in one position too long – bed sores begin this way). We then try to lift the head off the pillow (this weighs between 10–12lbs!!!). This action done regularly has caused a condition known as Torticollis or wry neck (misalignment of a vertebra in the neck), an extremely painful condition that prevents you from moving your head for quite some time.

The Safe Way

Is to sleep on your sides or your back. To break yourself of this very unsafe habit (as I had to), see Subconscious Mind.

4. Head position in bed

Believe it or not, it is important to be aware of your head position in bed. When it is regularly on the pillow nose up it is in hyper extension or nose down (chin on chest) – hyper flexion. Again not a particularly drastic habit but as we have learned when you sleep your body goes into dead weight mode so the head becomes heavy in the position it is in. This habit may be sufficient to damage the nerves in the neck that supply the head, shoulders, arms and hands because you have crushed the vertebra that way.

The Safe Way

Try to keep the neck in the neutral position therefore there is no strain on the vertebra and therefore no chance of crushing the nerves.

5. Pillows – the right one for you

If you stand in front of a mirror the distance between your ear and the outer most part of your shoulder is the height your pillow should be as this will keep your cervical spine (neck) in neutral when you are lying down. Too soft; it sags, and the head drops into lateral hyper flexion, too high it forces the head up into lateral hyper extension, both will harm the body if done habitually.

6. Beds – Life expectancy... When to turn. Sagging mattresses

I am informed by a bed manufacturer that you should change your bed or at least your mattress every ten years. And to prevent sagging in the middle, rotate the mattress or turn it over monthly. But please do it with your partner, not on your own! If you live on your own and have a double bed then sleep on one side one week then the other the next and get a friend to help you turn it over/around.

Personally, I feel that water beds are by far the best choice, for many reasons: they never need turning, they relieve pressure areas, are good for asthmatics, some forms of eczema sufferers, etc., since there is no material mattress for the bed bugs to live in (this is what aggravate these conditions) In addition, you don't have to replace them every ten years. You might want to research them? They do independent water mattresses in-cased in the one double bed, so when your partner turns over it doesn't disturb you. They are also fitted with independent heaters so you can choose how warm you want to be, in your half of the bed!

7. Making a bed
Please don't lean over by bending your back to pull the covers over both sides at once. This bending twisting movement habit is weakening the lower back, which over time with all the other habits, will cause the lower back to become inflamed. If your bed has sheets, do *not* bend over, the action of bending your back while pushing with your hands puts unnecessary strain on the lower back.

The Safe Way
Beds with sheets – go down on one knee to tuck them in. Beds with duvets do one side at a time, bending your knees not your back to do this action.

8. Cleaning teeth/face shaving etc.
We all do these every day, some twice a day – wow what a habit! If it's good then great. Chances are it's not. We all load the toothbrush and lean towards the sink in case it drips off the brush/out of our mouths so the straight posture has now

got a slight incline. Next time you do this stand up then place your palm of the hand on your low back and then bend forward as you would to clean your teeth/shave feel the pressure on the low back? This is creating the bending/straightening effect which if we were metal we would eventually snap! (See Carrie's rule of ninety).

The Safe Way

Stand with feet wider than hips bend the knees slightly and keep the back straight. There is little or no pressure on the back doing this then when you are ready to spit lean forward in this position and after return to the knee bent position. This has the added bonus of firming your thighs!

Note: if you are in the habit of putting your mouth under the tap to rinse your mouth – DON'T – this is a bending and twisting action that will cause problems in the end. Use a glass it saves your back and is far more hygienic!

9. Getting dressed/undressed

If I could instil just one change in the _world_ it would be this one! If you read through you will see just how much common sense this is…

It seems madness to be told how to get dressed and undressed but this is probably one of the most devastating bad habits going… why? Because most of us have been taught (by peers/parents) to stand up to put on the lower garments e.g., pants, socks, trousers, etc. and taught usually before we can stand up properly ourselves!

Then once learned we grow in this habit and when in a rush to get dressed we end up dancing and stumbling around with the occasional fall (hopefully onto the bed or nearby chair!). This action which was taught to us as a child is carried with us throughout the *whole* of our lives and seems fine while we are young enough to have our balance and the muscles to stop you when you begin to falter (fall) *but* as you get older the other bad habits you have developed all your life have not only made your back weak but also and probably worse, the muscles in your legs that are needed to stop you falling are now non-existent because of their lack of use!!!

UK Health statistics state that 72% of *ALL* people over 65 will be hospitalised, require some form of surgery as a result of falling and a good proportion of those falls will have been caused by falling when getting dressed!!!

The Safe Way

If you observe a toddler trying to dress for the first time (see pic on next page), they will automatically sit down to put on their socks, trousers, etc. yet as parents we make them stand up and alter this action to the habit we have been taught by our parents… it doesn't make it right!

Put very simply you cannot fall, wobble or dance around from a sitting position.

To dress: Sit on a chair/floor, feed the legs of the trousers/pants, etc., through each foot and THEN stand up firmly on *two* feet. Therefore, I urge you to get dressed/undressed for your lower body from a sitting position so you *Don't* become a statistic. If you change no other habit, **please *change this one*** – you won't regret it! In addition, pass it on to others…

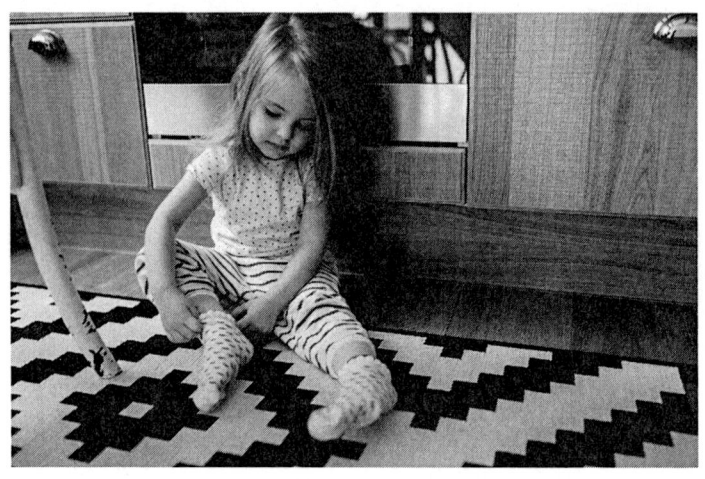

10. Putting on/taking off shoes/boots

Most people will stand up and slot their feet into their shoes or boots to put them on and then either lift their leg to pull them fully on or bend forward to pull them on. Bending puts unnecessary pressure on the low back, while the twisting movement needed when lifting one leg means the spine is put in a dangerous position. This repeated action will weaken the lower spine. Taking them off we usually put one toe in front of the other heel and lever them off. This is an exceptionally bad habit, not just because it is so regularly performed but because it employs only the very low back when this action is done, if the vertebra is disturbed it can cause all manner of problems including sciatica!

The Safe Way

Sit down to put them on/take them off! If you put on shoes from *sitting* you can bend forward flexing the spine in a safe way and use fingers/shoehorns to assist in getting them to fit. When taking them off again sit down and then you can put one foot in front of the other to remove shoes/boots from because now you will be using your upper thigh muscles *not* your back.

11a. Getting in/out of car

Most people who drive will leave the right foot anchored outside the car while lifting the left foot to put inside the car. Then, to manoeuvre the body to be able to sit down you swing the body around. This puts a twisting shearing action on the (low to mid-back) lumbar thoracic area if repeated will weaken this area.

The Safe Way

Open the car door, turn so your bottom is facing the inside of the car seat. Gently lower your bottom onto the seat. Then keeping knees and feet tight together (do not let them splay apart) lift the knees and feet together and bring them both into the car. **To alight** – simply reverse the process.

11b. Getting in/out of car

Shutting the car door when inside the car. It is important that you don't open the car door too wide since sitting in the car means you will have to lean to grab the door and pull it towards you. This habit can and (take my word for it) has caused misalignment of the spine creating severe pain and discomfort.

The Safe Way

When getting in the car ensure the door is not open to its widest and have your hand on the handle as you begin to sit *correctly* into the car, this way when you take your legs into the car the door is within easy reach. A great habit to get into!

Remember…

**It's not WHAT action you do…
It's HOW you do it.**

If how you do an action is 'quicker and easier'… it's usually *wrong*!!!

12. Standing (1) – weight unevenly on feet

This is probably one of the most commonly done habits done by nearly everyone! It is really bad for you since it places all your body's weight over one hip while at the same time it bends the lower spine away from the leg you are transferring your weight on. Repetition of this habit will cause the spine to form a J-shape at the bottom, obviously, this will load the body's weight unevenly on the lower spine and hips and is an accident waiting to happen. This can cause nerve pain pathway pain (known as referral) as pressure is put abnormally on the spinal discs this presses on the nerve and creates symptoms/pain along its pathway (and not necessarily in the back) e.g., sciatica.

12a. Standing (2)/walking with feet ten to two

If I use an analogy for this habit, it may be clearer for you to understand – if you get on a bike and you turn the handlebars right, the wheels turn right and so you move to the right, similarly turning left has the same reaction. So why point your feet outward when you intend to walk forward?

Surprisingly enough, this action does an awful lot of damage to your body, by way of compensation. It will cause incorrect loading of your body's weight over the joints chiefly the ankle and knee. Chances are if you are standing like this you will be walking like this too and this will be creating a shearing effect at the knee particularly, and if you are heavy-set this will wear the bones at the wrong angle which over time will create problems and pain (usually diagnosed as arthritis and or necessitating a knee replacement). In addition, this way of walking means that the arms are unable to swing normally by your side as you walk so your upper body will again compensate by swinging them from your shoulders so the whole posture has this gentle upper body swagger about it.

The Safe Way

Get an honest friend to observe how you are walking, or better still get them to make a video of you so you can see for yourself. If you feel you are not walking the correct way then you will need to retrain yourself to walk with your feet pointing forwards (heel to toe) you may need to refer to chapter five – to find out how to change a habit.

If by correcting this you find you have aches/pain elsewhere in the body – please seek help/treatment for this as this may very well be the reason you opted to change your gait (style of walking). This bad habit can be a result of a low back problem, ill-fitting shoes, or an unhealed/badly healed foot/knee/ankle injury. Not only will it make you walk wrongly but it will cause postural compensation elsewhere in your spine (for example rounding of shoulders)

13. Sitting at a desk/computer

This is a habit that the majority of us do without even thinking about it. Unfortunately, this includes those of you who are lucky enough to have 'risk assessments' at your workplace!! For although they have assessed your workstations, that was most likely in the days of computers, *not* laptops or tablets and technology is superseding these modern machines almost daily. In addition, and more importantly, they assessed your workplace *not* you! And it is *you* that I am concerned with/for. It is how you sit at your desk and what you do whilst you are sitting at it that concerns me.

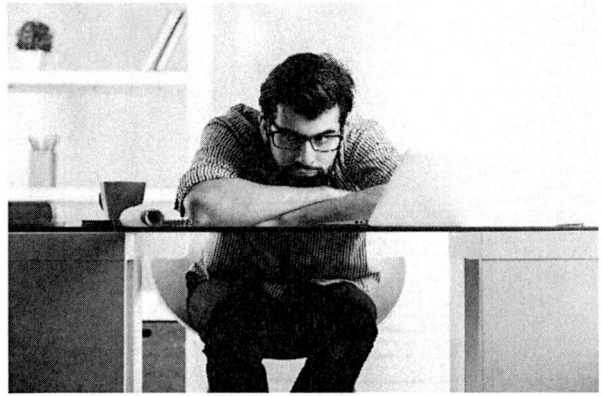

Wrong posture! Person's head and upper torso forward, shoulders are rounded.

It is vital that you break this bad habit since you may spend as much as eight hours per weekday in this position. The man above clearly demonstrates the bad postural position when we get involved in the work that we are doing. It's so easy to do… even now I find myself correcting myself regularly and I am supposed to know the correct posture! A question for you… do you remember how much the head weighs? Answer: 1/10th of your body weight, so if you weigh ten stones then your head weighs one stone! Therefore, if your posture means your head is forward, rather than correct posture i.e., the weight of the head is evenly distributed front and back then all that strain goes on your neck and upper spine! Let me talk about the various bad positions people get into just sitting at a desk, these pictures demonstrate a few of the problem areas. On the previous page, the man at the desk clearly demonstrates the harmful positions people who concentrate can end up in. Pressure will be mainly on low, middle and neck spine, so altogether a bad habit to have.

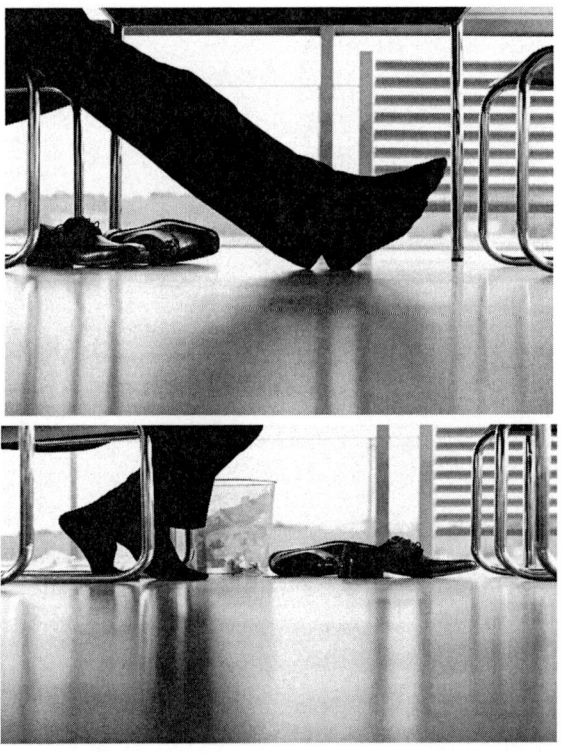

Sitting with your feet tucked under your chair or out in front of you causes the body to either, rock forward (anteriorly tilting the pelvis) or rock backward (posterior tilt to the pelvis). Over time this will crush the lumbar spinal discs.

And as for the so-called postural chair, I would like to pick it up and throw it as far as I can!! If you look at the picture you will see the lower back is forced into an indent position this is the same result as for tucking feet under a chair. In addition, this loads the hips and the bend at the knee shuts off the circulation to the lower leg/feet. You decide?

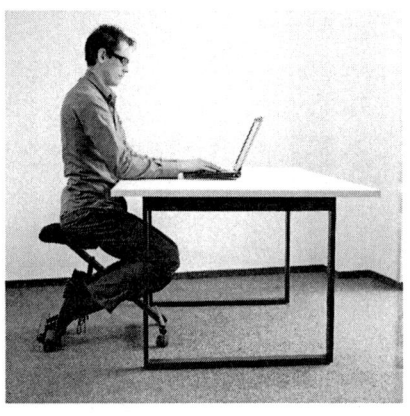

Postural chair – definitely a NO-NO!

The Safe Way

The ideal posture as demonstrated in chapter 7 is to sit up straight with your bottom into the base of the chair, your back on the back of the chair and your chin retracted back, your feet pointing forward and flat on the floor uncrossed (see Carrie's 'Rule of Ninety'). I have found (after many hours of trying) that the best way to change this very bad habit, is to definitely apply the 'how to change a bad habit' plus you will need additional help since this is a really difficult one to change… I suggest you set a timer for say five minutes (at first) and when it goes off stay *exactly* where you are, make a note of the position you are in, then correct it and use the how to change a habit policy, then reset your timer. You will undoubtedly be the same as me and fail miserably hundreds of times!! Take heart you can and will get there in the end. It's a real pain I know, but if you think about how many times you have to correct it you will then come to realise just how bad this habit of yours is and the damage you are permanently doing to your body.

This realisation will hopefully be the key to helping you correct it.

14. Tablets/laptops/mobile phones/hand-helds

Hmmm, whilst we are on the subject of computers. The picture below, right is typical of people today, young or old, totally engrossed in what they are doing oblivious to the harm they may be caused from bad posture not to mention the possibility of putting themselves in grave danger from not looking where they are going! This is the same action when using a laptop since it will encourage your head to tilt down straining the base of the neck, the body recognises this strain and lays down protective layering at this point forming an unsightly fatty lump (on left) known as a dowager's hump.

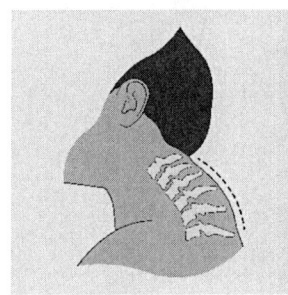
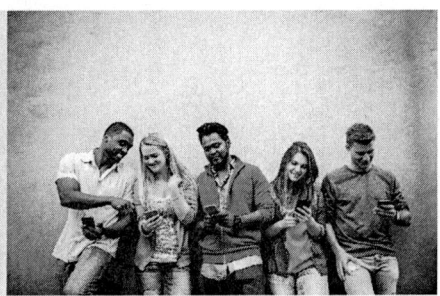

The Safe Way

If you really can't wait to read/write a text where it is safe, then hold the phone/tablet up at eye height, this does two things; it allows your eyes to have peripheral vision to be able to notice danger more easily (it is not a substitute for not texting in the first place); it corrects your bad postural bent head that creates the ugly dowagers hump, neck disc compression that can lead to symptoms such as carpal tunnel symptoms, a win-win situation all round. When using a laptop, raise it up by placing it on something like a cushion on your lap, this brings the machine up to eye height, keeping the head in the correct neutral posture.

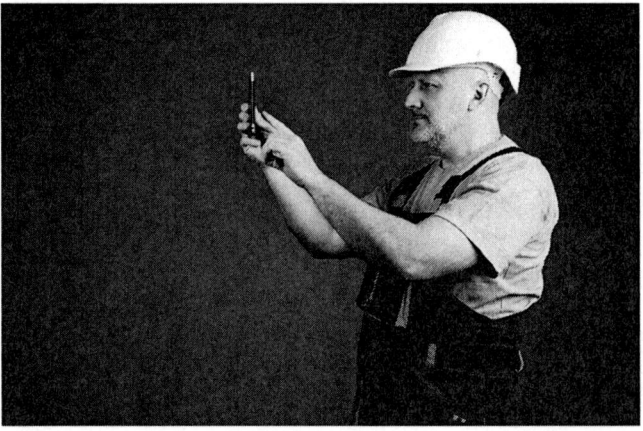

Hold the item up to eye height rather than bend heavy head forward putting strain on the neck.

15. Lying on the sofa/couch

My advice for this bad habit is to try to get out of it altogether! This is because you will undoubtedly lie on the sofa the same way = repetitively (to watch TV usually) and more often than not, use the armrest as your pillow as this is too high and unyielding it puts your neck and spine at risk! If it is because you are tired, go to bed!

The Safe Way

There really is no safe way to 'lie' on a sofa that has been designed and tested for sitting on.

16. Sitting on a sofa

Seems silly to mention how people sit on a sofa but you would be surprised at how many bad backs are caused because of bad habits and ill-fitting sofas. The most common very damaging habit mainly done by women is sitting on the sofa with your legs tucked up underneath you, leaning to one side (on the arm) of the sofa. This puts huge pressure on your spine and forces it out of its natural straight shape. When done habitually, the spinal disc will eventually be crushed on that side, resulting in nerve pathway inflammation and pain (see spine on front cover). In addition, if you are carrying excess weight the time frame for this to occur is much less!

Unfortunately, manufacturers do not take into consideration people's height, therefore if you are short or tall you are probably not sitting correctly on a sofa because you will have had to adjust your sitting position to accommodate it, rather than the other way around!

Be warned modern sofas with low backs, offer NO support for your head/neck at all! In addition, cheap sofa's, in particular, seem to have a limited shelf life, leaving sagging springs and cushions that put your spine at risk.

The Safe Way

Sit squarely on the sofa (see the rule of ninety) if you need extra support either get a recliner or alternatively a foot stool. If you are short, try to ensure you have cushions at the back of you (I have two!), these allow you to put your knee crease at the edge of the sofa and your feet on the floor, conversely, if you are tall try to remove cushions to obtain the same result. If the cushions don't plump up anymore – time to buy a new sofa!

17. Recliners

If you are thinking of getting a recliner chair, then please consider this. It is important to ensure the action of putting it into the recliner position is able to be achieved with ease, so many I have tried, you have to fight with it in order for it to recline and then when you want it upright again, you have to be some sort of gymnast to be able to do this! In addition, *don't buy* the ones where the back of the recliner leans back at an obtuse angle, this puts strain on your lower back putting you at a severe disadvantage in this chair if you want to watch TV/DVDs, etc.

The Safe Way

When purchasing a recliner, ensure that the device (handle or remote) allows the recline to be carried out with ease. In addition, note the chair back itself must remain in the upright position throughout.

18. Running – road cambers

Apart from the obvious; correct fitting, road worthy shoes, and correct technique… the 'unobvious' postural habit is running the same way (route) all the time. Should there be a camber on the road, your body will be thrown that way too (OK for short or occasional runs), really bad if marathon training (prolonged lengthy runs) because of the obtuse angle obtained, in addition to the neck.

The Safe Way

Ensure that you change the running direction daily. Go one way one day and reverse it the next and keep those feet pointed forwards.

19. Shoes – Fashion, trainers, flatties, platforms, wedges

Wearing ill-fitting shoes just for fashion is a recipe for disaster and creates postural problems; for example, if your shoes are too high, they will tilt you forward so your body will automatically lean back to balance you this puts unnatural strain on your spine, tight shoes will make you walk differently and on a different part of the foot (to get out of pain), etc., this will have repercussions on the posture. Hard to believe but 'flatties' discourage the natural arch in your foot and encourage the person to drag their feet, both of these are damaging to your posture. Platforms and wedges prevent correct foot movement (part of the walking cycle) putting strain on the knees, hips and lower back as the body tries to compensate to obtain/correct the walking mechanism.

The Safe Way

I am not saying you cannot wear heels, just be sensible. As for 'flatties', wedges and platforms, the sooner they go out of fashion, the better!

21. The long and short of it – 1

This refers to the height of people and how it affects their posture. I am informed sound waves travel best horizontally, therefore, do not travel well upwards or downwards. It goes without saying then that people who are taller or shorter than average will find it difficult to hear what is being said when in a group of people or if the person they are speaking to is quietly spoken. The taller person will repeatedly bend their heads low in an attempt to bring their ears as close to the 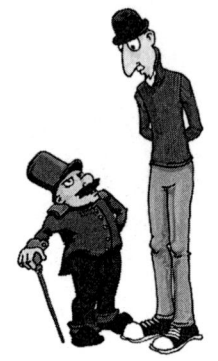 sound waves as possible, whilst the shorter person will extend their head (backwards) to try to catch the sound waves. This repetitive action will crush neck discs!

The Safe Way

In order to be able to hear the sound waves easier, place one foot in front of you so it is nearest the group and then take.

One step back, your legs are now splayed. Rest the body on the back foot*, this takes your head further away from the group and allows the waves to dissipate enabling you to hear better whilst at the same time maintaining your position in the crowd/group and preventing your head from moving out of 'postural neutral'. *NB – vary the back foot.

22. <u>The long and short of it – 2</u>

Short people have a problem with sitting on normal chairs/sofas as their legs don't bend where the cushions/chair seat ends, so in order for them to look as though they are sitting comfortably, they must either slump in the chair so their knees bend at the end of the chair or stack a whole lot of cushions behind their back, with chairs when they are sitting with their bottoms correctly in the back their legs are swinging in the breeze (they have said this makes them feel like a child so they tend to hook them around the front legs of the chair – a definite No-No). This will be particularly true when they sit on a bar stool as the footrest tends to be quite low down.

Tall people, when seated on a chair have their knees some distance from the edge of the seat this causes discomfort and puts unnecessary pressure on the back of their upper legs.

23. Sitting on a breakfast/bar stool

The main problem with this bad habit is of course the way you sit on the stool. And this applies to any stool to be candid. When we sit on a stool two things happen… Firstly, the body realises there is no/very low back to the chair so will automatically try to balance as best we can, trying to keep back straight in line with gravity. Secondly, the body will compensate in trying to keep the back straight by tipping the pelvis forward this means the top half of your body will tilt backwards slightly to keep the body perpendicular. This action crushes all the lower lumbar vertebral discs. If you are regularly sitting on a stool (I am thinking here of a lot of therapists) you will automatically take up this position – I speak here with HUGE experience! This extremely bad habit will cause a devastating effect on your lower spine and their discs that may be irreversible! So please take heed of the safe way.

The Safe Way

When you sit on the stool ensure that your bottom is right at the back of it, push the lower back downwards, at this point you can now straighten your back (in line with gravity). However, you need to hold this position whilst you are on the stool, this is not easy to do and when you relax you will tilt the pelvis forwards thus putting strain on the spine.

24. <u>Moulded seats</u> (Arghh!)

I am talking here of the sort that is designed to stack up quickly (see picture below). Normally found in scout huts, village halls, etc., Note the rounding of the chair, where the bottom sits, prevents the lower back from obtaining 90 degrees. Also, the back rest shape prevents the upper body from obtaining 90 degrees. The line indicates where the person's upper body would be if they leaned back on the chair.

The Safe Way

Obviously, the safest way is not to sit on this type of chair at all!!! However, if you have to sit on them, ensure that you roll up your cardy/scarf/coat/even handbag to put at the back of you (in the base of the back) so it acts as a support to keep your posture at the ninety degrees it needs to be.

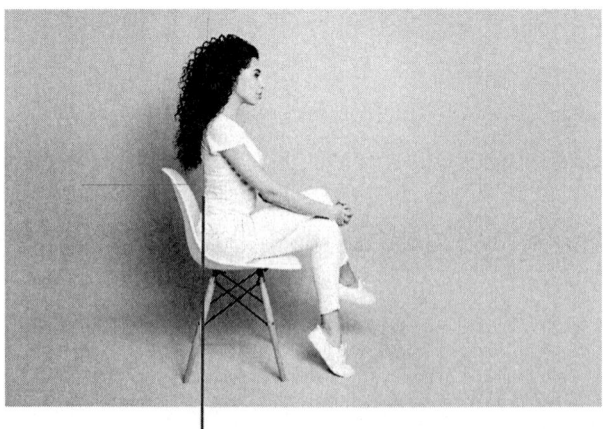

25. Carrying a ruck sack

The ruck sack can be a man's best friend when it comes to carrying heavy things. However, if it is not fitted correctly i.e., too loose/tight or put on correctly, it can do more harm than good (picture below left). When putting on the rucksack do not pick it up with one hand and 'sling it' over your shoulder, this twists the spine with load and is an accident waiting to happen. It is not cool to sling it over just one shoulder overloading that shoulder and then the bodyweight compensates for that one-sided load by moving the body to try and equal the weight.

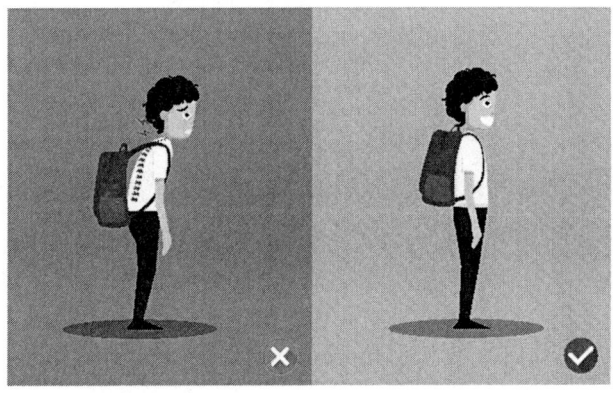

The Safe Way

(Picture right above) To fit the rucksack correctly the straps should be tightened so that the bottom of the sack sits mid-back. Not resting on your bottom. The most important thing to remember about a rucksack is that it has *two* straps… therefore it is important that you use them! When fully laden/heavy, try to find a table/wall/surface the height of your back/bottom, then correctly lift (back straight, knees bent) the rucksack and place on that surface with straps facing you, now feed your arms into the straps and gently ease the body of the rucksack into position on your back. Practice makes perfect and you'll be doing it just as quickly as you used to!

Remember – if it's quicker and easier to do an action – it's usually wrong!

It's not what you action you do, it's the way that you do it

26. Gardening/bending over to pick up something

This is one of the worst bad habits for creating problems. Once you know how to do it correctly just take a look around your neighbourhood and see how many folks are gardening/bending wrongly (picture left below). The majority of us have copied the way we have seen our parents bend and then we pass that action onto our children! When a person stands with their legs straight and bends their back forward, it puts amazing repetitive strain on the lower back remaining in this position for some time will add to the problem especially if it is with a load for example pulling up stubborn plants, picking up a heavy or awkward object. This habit is usually combined with another… see No. 27

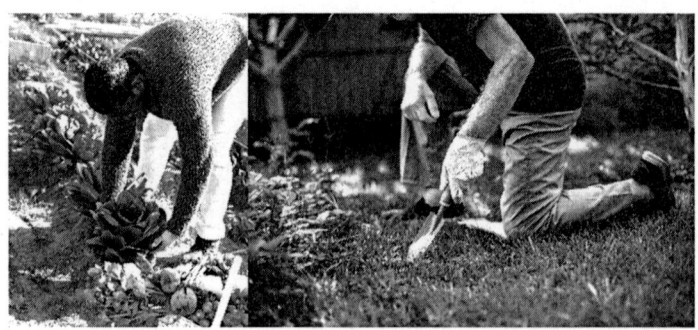

The Safe Way

Is to keep the back straight and kneel on one knee (pictured right), you can use the upper bent knee to rest your arm on whilst you garden. In addition, in this position you can change the knee you are bending on to give a wider range of gardening movement without even getting up!

27. <u>Kneeling on both knees (to do an action)</u>

This is on a par with one of the *worst* bad habits I can identify, worse still there are companies selling gardening kneeling stools that encourage and sanctify this bad habit, it might make it easier but it isn't the safe way. Kneeling on both knees and then doing an action (e.g., gardening, scrubbing floors, changing baby's nappy etc.) will put a huge strain directly on the lower back, especially if you have both hands engaged in doing an action e.g., changing a baby's nappy (see below). If you are kneeling on the floor resting on one hand using the other to work with, this action

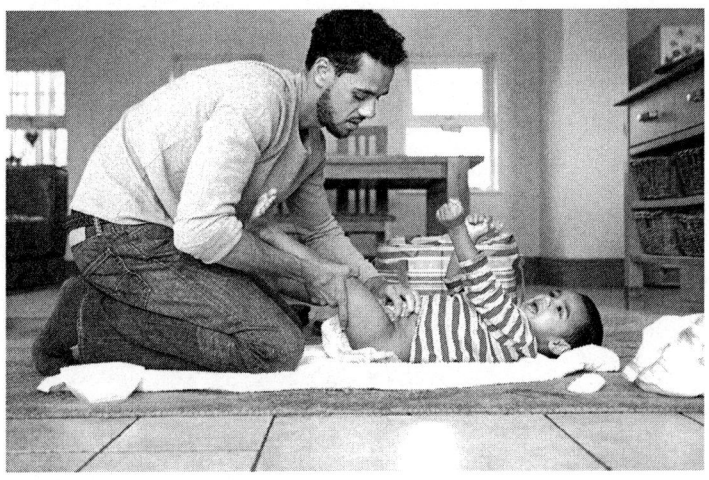

twists the spine and usually done in the same way, since you are either right or left-handed using a tool, brush, etc., will cause repetitive twisting with a load on your spine; an accident waiting to happen in my experience.

The Safe Way

The safest way to do this is to adopt the same position as number 26, that is, one knee up and one down, this keeps the back/spine straight (picture right previous page).

28. Digging/shovelling

When digging there are two problems, pushing hard down using one leg and throwing the fork into the garden. The rebound that goes through the body can be very harmful. Using the same arm as you inevitably will throw the fork into the ground will create a repetitive action which is not too bad providing; the ground is not hard, the fork doesn't hit anything static, this causes a damaging jolt. Shovelling can be exceptionally damaging for your body. Normally people bend their backs to push in the shovel then using their arms (but mainly their backs) they lift the shovel head (see pictures next page), then leaving their feet where they are they twist the body (spine) and using a throwing action pull back and throw the contents of the shovel head to another area.

This repetitive action is an inevitable accident waiting to happen with your spine. You are putting a load on the end of the shovel, which ultimately puts excessive strain on the lower section of the middle vertebrae as well as the lower vertebrae.

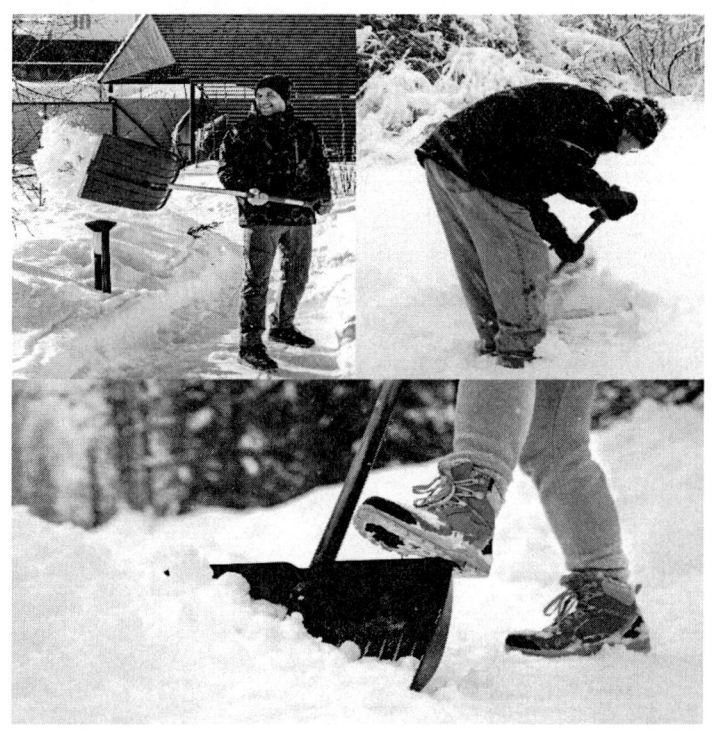

The Safe Way

Ensure that the garden has been well watered prior to starting to dig this will at least soften the ground to assist the fork going into the ground/soil. Always bend **both** knees to form a lunge position and keep the back straight when digging/shovelling, when there is loading, try to keep this as near to the body as possible and forward. Tilt the pelvis during the manoeuvre and keep both knees bent so you cannot use the low back. And don't be tempted to overload the shovel!

29. Pulling/pushing action e.g., sweeping, raking, hoeing, mowing the lawn, using a vacuum, mopping, etc.

The majority of people are unilateral in this action, that is they will use the dominant hand to 'work' with. The action used is a pushing or pulling action combined with a slight twist (spine) always to the same side, which when done regularly, will cause RSI (repetitive strain injury) at the very low back because the back is in the slightly bent position for long periods (see left picture below)

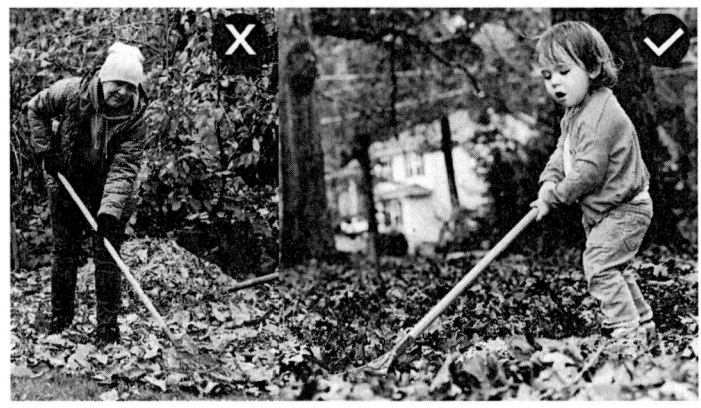

The Safe Way

For this new habit, the arms remain straight throughout holding the broom/rake, etc., for both pushing **or** pulling.

All the work is done by the front thigh muscles that use a rocking motion to move the upper body back and forth this movement is what does the sweeping/raking! The front leg is bent at the knee while the back leg remains straight (picture on right) the back is kept as straight as possible. This new way of doing this task will take a bit of getting used to but is essential for things like mopping the floor! (Note: the picture on previous page is of a *child* doing the correct action!)

30. <u>One-handed lifting actions</u>

For Example: using a watering can, carrying a handbag/laptop/briefcase, shopping, suitcase, etc. Most people will use their dominant hand to pick up/carry the load whilst the upper body is used to counterbalance the load. This puts an uneven strain on the spine both when picking up the object and when carrying it. Repeating this action will cause an imbalance in muscles and the muscle pull on the spine, particularly the lumbar section which in time will inevitably be an accident waiting to happen.

The Safe Way

Try not to overload what you are carrying and share the load, that is have two smaller bags of shopping one in each hand so that you remain balanced. Use a handbag/laptop that has a long strap that way you can carry it over one shoulder while the bag goes over the opposite hip, this leaves the hands free. When it comes to briefcases; it is best to alternate the hand you pick it up/carry it with. I have a little saying that might help you remember which hand you did what with… You *left* home but you will be *right* back = carry the briefcase to work in the *left* hand and on the return home journey, use the *right* hand. Ensure when shopping you have a bag in each hand of equal weight. This prevents you from using the upper body to counterbalance the imbalance. When using a watering can don't be tempted to overfill it. If you do, it will be very heavy to pick up and also even heavier to hold steady in one position for a length of time (while you water)… instead treat it as an exercise that you have to refill the can more often but remember to bend those knees and keep that back straight when you do, push the body up using the muscles in the front of the legs (quads). Suitcases pose another problem, try to take two smaller cases rather than one big one this will help equal out the load. Again, remember to lift correctly using the upper legs to push you upwards rather than the arms to jerkily lift the cases. Handbags are OK if they don't contain the kitchen sink! Ladies, trust me, you really don't need all that is in there – time for a decluttering perhaps? If you are a shoulder bag kinda gal, then ensure your strap is long enough to go over one shoulder and the bag over the opposite hip to equal the load, this leaves your hands free. But remember to alternate the shoulder/hip that you carry it on too.

31. <u>General lifting techniques</u>

When lifting anything, most people know they have to bend their knees BUT what they don't do is bend them enough! The majority of people bend their backs and I have noticed a lot of people sticking out their bottoms (See habit #32) and these habits allow the use of the lower part of the back to be employed in the lifting action!

The Safe Way

Most people know to keep heavy objects they are lifting as close to them as possible which helps prevent injuries. However, as you lift ensure the feet are pointing forward and at least hip width apart, bend the knees right down try to keep the feet *flat* on the floor, get as close to the object as possible, now tuck the pelvis under so it is tilted forwards, this action prevents you from using the lower back. Now for the important bit, using the muscles in the front of your leg (quads), grasp the object with your hands and push the body upwards using those big quad muscles all the while keeping your back as straight (perpendicular to gravity!) as possible.

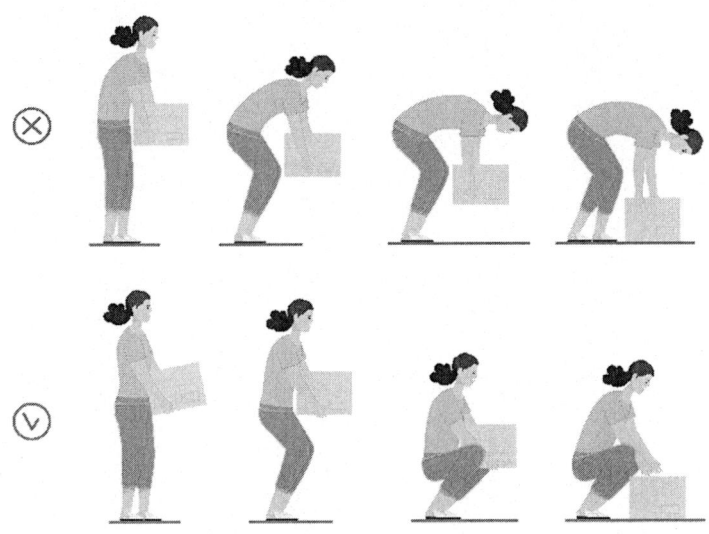

This action will ensure you lift correctly, protect your back in addition it will strengthen and tone your legs (bonus ☺).

32. Bending (in general)

This habit is essential to change since the majority of us in the western hemisphere do this (this is one of those actions we copy from one generation and pass on to another generation) This habit MUST be broken since in my experience, it is the major cause of later onset problems! The wrong way to bend even though knees are bent is shown below and should be avoided, even if it is to pick up a piece of paper/leaf/tie shoelaces etc.

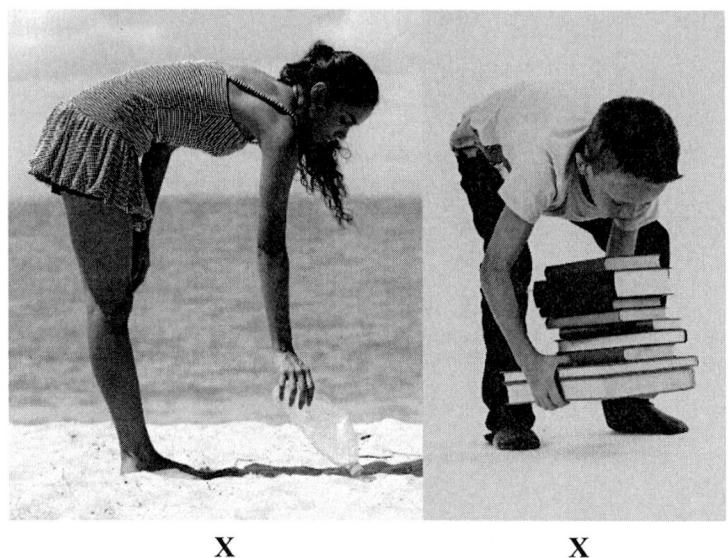

X   X

The Safe Way

The correct way is to split your feet so one foot is about 8–10 inches in front of the other and then drop the body between the two so your back is straight (see picture on next page). This allows complete stability, in addition, it means that you can now push up using those big thigh muscles and keeping your back straight as you do so. This will take practice but *please* use this method from now on.

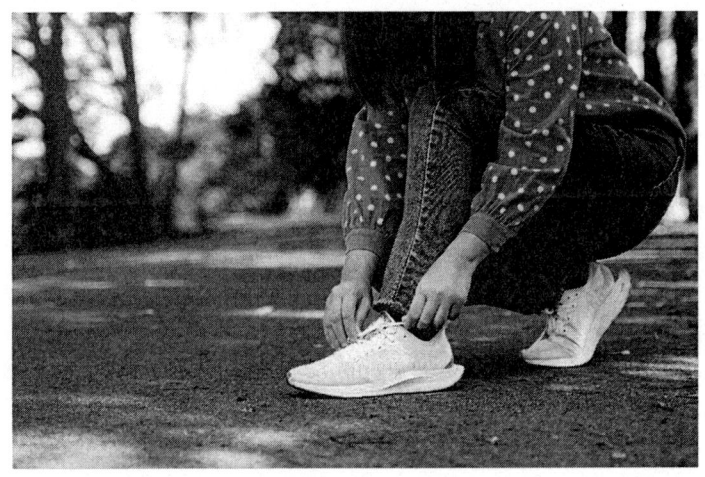

33. Putting things away/reaching a high shelf

The normal way that people achieve this action is to overstretch their arms whilst going on tiptoes. This action is usually accompanied by a load of some sort either to put something on the shelf or take it off or push or pull something open. It is common to favour the dominant hand making the stretch/strain always occurring on that side.

The Safe Way

Is to use a fold-away 'hop-up' they store flat and take no time at all to get out, it is just a question of getting into the new habit.

34. Putting things away low shelf/under the cupboard. Loading/unloading washing machine/under cupboard fridge/dishwasher/tumble drier etc.

All these actions use one of two movements; firstly the person rests on both knees whilst twisting their body to put things/reach to a low shelf. Secondly and more commonly, the person will bend over and twist their back whilst loading/unloading the dishwasher/washing machine, under cabinet fridge, etc., this is a really dangerous habit to get into since it puts the weight of the upper body, together with the weight of the load and the strain of the twist directly on the lower spine!

The Safe Way

Very simple – in order to go to the level of the 'machine', bend onto one knee and keep the back straight, see below.

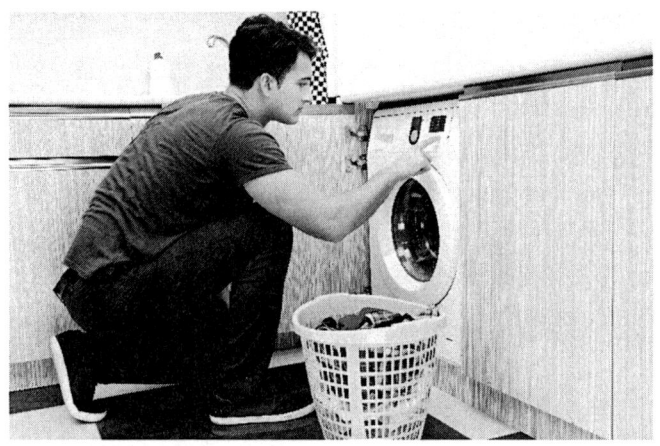

Remember – if it's quicker and easier to do an action – it's usually wrong!
It's not what action you do, it's how you do it.

35. Cleaning the car

This habit is one we all do. Most of us hold onto the car with one hand whilst bending our back over and twisting our spine to clean it with the other. Again this is usually done with the dominant hand, so repetition is a foregone conclusion. In addition, you will be exerting pressure with the cleaning hand and overreaching when doing the roof.

The Safe Way

For the lower half of the car, use the technique of bending on one knee (on a kneeling pad) or bop/crouch down. To do the upper half of the car, it is important to bend the knees and keep the back straight, I find if you spread your feet wide, keep the knees bent and back straight, in that position you can then move the upper body so it transfers the bodyweight from the left leg to the right leg, using the quad muscles. Using this action allows you to cover a larger area without having to move a great deal. To do the roof please use the 'hop up'.

36. Ladder work

Most people when up a ladder will hold on with one hand and 'do' the work with the other, no problem so far. However, they rest their knees on the ladder rungs to secure themselves and counterbalance the upper body movement. However, the knees need stability to hold them safely on the rung, in order to allow the body to lean away from the ladder, this puts pressure directly on the low back. So the longer you use the ladder the more strain is put on the lower back. Another common problem is overreaching, this not only puts one-sided strain on the body, but it is also seriously dangerous!

The Safe Way

Any ladder work done requires safety first. Someone to stay at the bottom to ensure the ladder doesn't slip. When at the top of the ladder affix yourself to something secure, then you can safely place your feet to the outsides of the ladder rung and stand on your two feet instead of leaning against the ladder with your knees, this way there is no strain on the back. As for the overreaching… it's simple, please don't take shortcuts just because you think it is easier to reach over rather than move the ladder! Remember if its quicker and easier….

37. Worktop preparations/washing up/bench-work

Speaking of leaning, people who use a worktop to work on have a bad habit of resting their hip/tummy/waist area against the worktop whilst working on the surface. This action puts direct pressure on the low back.

The Safe Way

Stand slightly away from the worktop and then slightly bend the knees and keep your pelvis in neutral this means you will be at the right height and the knees bent position will allow you to maintain a straight back essential to prevent low back strain.

38. Answering the phone

When using the phone correctly there is no problem. However, it is when the phone is held between the shoulder and the ear that the bad habit occurs. The person will normally perform this action on the same side (usually dominant) and if it is a regular habit will shorten that side's muscles and overstretch the other side. These are major muscles that contribute to the neck/shoulder movement so imperative they remain equal.

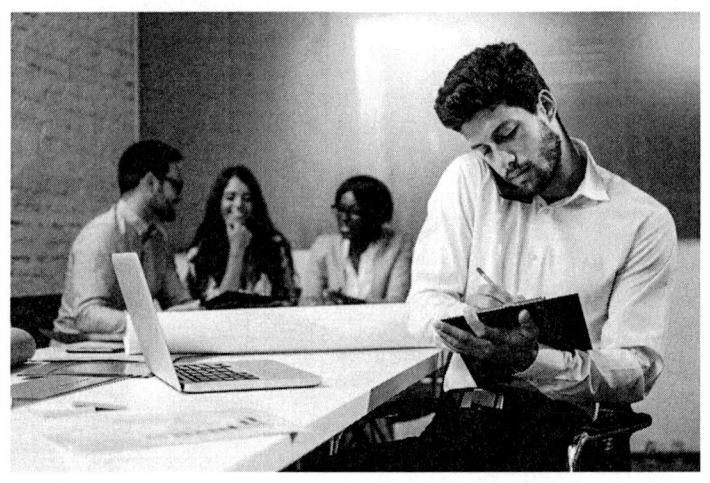

The Safe Way

Obviously, the best way is to hold the phone to the ear. If this is not possible, then if you are doing a receptionist type job it is the responsibility of the workplace to supply you with headphones to enable you to have both hands free to write notes, type, etc., if you need your hands to write, etc., put the phone on speaker phone for the duration needed.

39. <u>Multi-tasking</u>

The problem with multi-tasking is that the brain is thinking about too many things at once and the last thing it will be considering is your posture! (i.e., how you are doing all these actions!) The mind is racing and concentrating on asking the body to do the many tasks you are demanding of it. Believe me when I say I have done the 'multi-tasking malarkey' and ended up either making a mess of the thing I was doing or injuring myself in my haste to get it done (Pic below)! Multi-tasking encourages quick fixes.

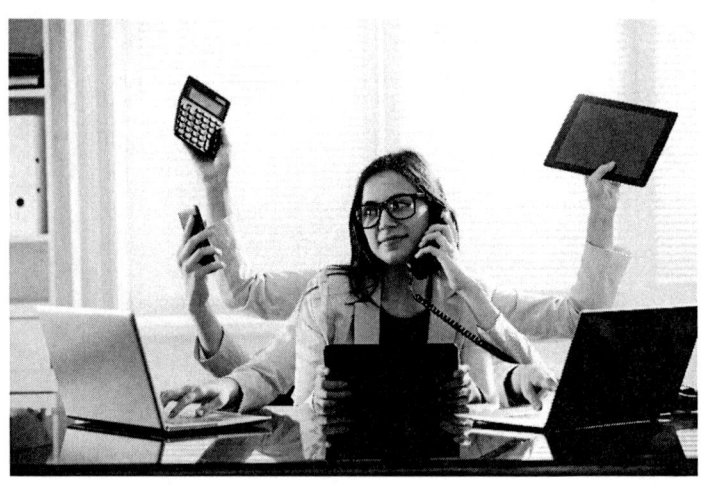

The Safe Way

The safest way is to put multitasking on the back burner for a while. Instead initially, you will need to prioritise the tasks so that you can do them one at a time and do them safely and well. I realise in this 'fast modern world' time is of the essence, but trust me when I say it will take much longer in the end with the added problem that you will unquestionably be creating, rehearsing and putting into action all the bad habits you have learned so far in order to accomplish so many things in such a short time, and this will cost your body dearly! Now, I say initially because don't despair... all is not lost! Once you have corrected the majority of your bad habits, and the new way of doing actions have taken over and become your good habits, your multi-tasking can resume because you will be doing each action correctly *and* with speed (as I now do). It just takes time so please don't be impatient, it has taken you a long time to acquire the bad habits you now possess so it will take a while to change them all.

Remember – if it's quicker and easier to do an action – it's usually wrong!
It's not what action you do, it's how you do it.

40. <u>Overhead Work</u>

The majority of us use a ladder, hop up, chair, etc., to obtain as near as we can to the ceiling/top then stretch our arms to the rest of the way usually with an object in our hands to 'do' the task. It may be a light object for e.g., a light bulb/paintbrush, or it could be heavy e.g., a hedge cutter. The heavier the object the more strain on the upper part of the spine/back (mainly between the shoulder blades). If you are reaching beyond your stretch with a load, you are putting excessive strain on your spine. In addition, when doing overhead work for any length of time your head will be in the overextended position, squeezing the bones in the neck (cervical vertebrae) and the spongy shock absorbers that go in between them (discs). Therefore, regular workers will be compressing this part which is very dangerous since the main nerve supply to the head and face lie in the upper part of the neck and the main nerve supply to the shoulders and arms/hands is in the lower part of the neck and between the shoulder blades. If these vertebrae get damaged, they will press on those nerves and pain will be felt where the nerve pathway goes. Normally we just look up, and it is this action that crushes the vertebrae and the discs.

The Safe Way

If you are doing regular overhead work, the first thing you must learn is how to look up correctly. In order to protect your neck – with your head in neutral, that is the chin is directly in front, not pointing up or down; then bring the chin back as far as far as it will go (as if making a double chin); now in this position look up at the ceiling, you will notice that you can now obtain a better range of movement without putting excessive pressure on the vertebrae or discs (though over time they will inevitably wear).

41. Painting… Fences, walls, etc.

Most people tend to use a paintbrush to put on as much paint and to cover as much of the area as possible without having to move. As such we tend to overstretch the 'paintbrush' arm which is usually done with the dominant arm. This puts strain on that shoulder girdle, blade, upper spine and neck. If this is a one-off task you will certainly get away with doing it like you always have done. However, if you have a lot of painting to do or it is your regular job then you will be creating upper body one-sided repetitive strain. Most people will go on both knees to paint the lower half and to stand on a stool and overstretch to reach the top part.

The Safe Way

It might seem a little arduous at first but the best thing to do is treat it like you are doing a form of exercise and to *praise* yourself well after you have achieved your goal (painted the fence etc.) so, to do the lower work ensure you kneel correctly that is one knee up and one down this keeps the back (spine) straight, and to make it even easier, change to the other knee while you are still kneeling down to give you a wider range of painting area. To do the top ensure you have steps that allow you good access. Failing that, I'm afraid it is just a question of not being lazy, it just means that you have to move the steps/ladder more often (but as I said if you think of it as being your exercise burning off the calories and toning up the muscles or, as the late Sir Wogan would say, 'fighting the flab', you will be OK).

42. Ironing

Make ironing fun and tone those flabby thighs while you do your chores correctly. We all know how you normally stand to iron so enough said about that, however, if you sit down to do it you will be grounding your lower half and this means your upper half will be twisting, putting strain on the low spine.

The Safe Way

Here's the best way to protect your back as well as give you a good workout. Set the board a little lower than you normally would, this prevents the (ironing) shoulder from being held in the raised up lifted position, now stand four inches away, feet wider than hip width apart and pointing forward. Now slightly bend the knees and keep the back straight, in this position hold the iron *but* instead of using the arm to push the iron back and forth, hold the iron still and transfer the upper body weight from one knee to the other in a swaying (rocking) motion, this action will move the iron back and forth whilst at the same time work the upper thighs!

43. Housework/Cleaning

This is a task we all do on a regular basis and most of us want to get it done in double quick time as it is not our favourite pastime! The actions we did at the very start of doing the housework will be the ones we continue to do throughout. Chores that will create more bad habits than any other since it is one that is done for a long, long time!

Therefore, it is imperative to do the actions correctly so that this repetitious vocation be done correctly *all* the time.

We all know how 'we' do the actions so it might be prudent to just go through the correct actions for doing the various chores. Introducing 'The Housework Workout!' Instead of treating the housework as a chore, think of it as a workout! Toning muscles, doing the chores while protecting your spine. How cool is that?

a) Sweeping/Cleaning floors using a mop/vacuuming.

As this is a one-sided action it is imperative that it be done correctly as it will be straining one side constantly. Therefore, hold the mop as normal but use the feet to propel you forward and back rather than your arms/shoulders, i.e., keep arms still and propel the mop forward by stepping forward then step back to return the mop. I agree it is arduous *but* it will keep your body safe, strengthen and tone the upper leg muscles *and* burn off those calories – bonus!

b) Polishing furniture (as for car).

Again, this is usually a dominant-sided action and although it is not always safe to use the other hand it would be beneficial if you could learn to do the action with both hands (most people have never tried!) when doing the action try to get as close to the object as possible and make small circular movements rather than larger ones and don't over-stretch, move closer. Also try to polish anticlockwise as well as clockwise. This will use different muscles, of the shoulder girdle.

c) **Scrubbing floors/cleaning skirting etc.**

Try to get used to doing any floor work/actions using one knee up and one down and alternating them, this maintains a straight back while protecting the lower spine. This will use and tone muscles you don't normally use.

d) **Overhead work.**

Use an extendible feather duster to clean coving, overhead lighting and ceilings. Don't be tempted to overreach, use a hop-up or steps again working those muscles.

e) **Moving furniture.**

Housework is renowned for being done by women though I am very much aware that there are more and more house-husbands regardless of gender, moving furniture on your own is a no-no! Even worse is putting your hip up against the object to assist/add weight to move the object, this is one of the most dangerous actions since the twist/strain is directly on the lowest lumbar vertebra. I have corrected more of these vertebrae from doing this type of action than most!

f) **Making beds.**

Most of us these days have duvet covers, very few have blankets but regardless of either, the action is the same. Usually, you lean over to 'flick' the sheets/duvet cover to make up the other side. This action means that you will be bending and twisting with a jerking motion, a habit that you really must get out of. The correct way is to do one side at a time and go around to each side, ensuring that you bend the knees to keep the back straight to tuck it in. When pulling the duvet/sheet up, do not be tempted to lean the legs up against the bed as this puts direct strain on the lower spine.

g) **<u>Hanging out the washing</u>**.

As this is a severely repetitive action you must ensure that every time you bend to pick up a piece of laundry you fully bend the knees (bop down) and use your thighs to push you back up to straight. This is a fantastic workout for those thighs ☺.

44. <u>Nodding off (when seated)</u>

As we now know, the head weighs $1/10^{th}$ bodyweight. That weight should be evenly distributed between the front of the chest and the back, spreading the load equally. Just bear this fact in mind as you read on… The habit of nodding off when seated is one that can cause you real problems with your neck/shoulders/arms. I have seen this habit done so regularly by the young and old alike. The elderly has a habit of nodding off in an armchair after lunch when that sneaky nap just kinda creeps up on them and they end up having 'forty winks' while both young and old tend to take a 'power nap' on trains, planes and the underground, where people have got up very early or are bored on a long journey.

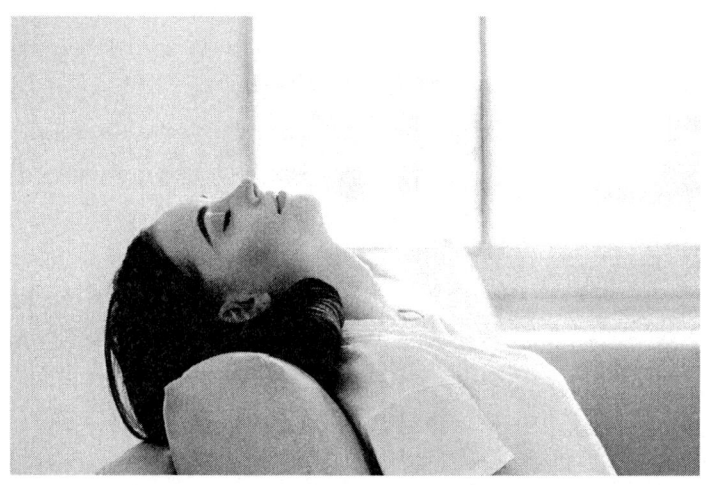

Heads going too far back or too far forward damage the neck.

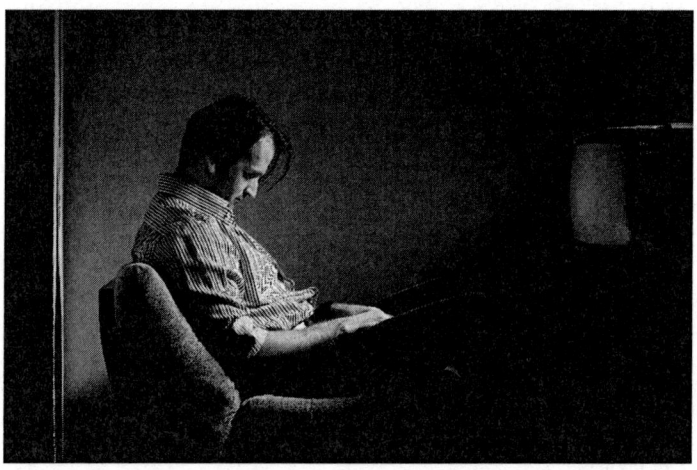

This action allows the weight of their head to drop forward/crash back unsupported, bouncing around with every movement of the vehicle. Sitting in this position your head is either all in front so the weight is forward and the strain is on the back of the spine at the neck, or all at the back crushing the spine in the neck. Now because the brain knows you need to be aware of your surroundings (for protection) and that is not supposed to be asleep at this time, your subconscious takes over, the longer you sleep the more strain on your neck and so if/when there is a loud noise or disruption to the familiar noises, your subconscious alerts you, causing you to jerk awake. It is this jerk that can cause a whiplash effect and quite possibly cause a misaligned vertebra. This will cause pain in the neck and shoulders and if bad enough the nerve pathway can radiate into the arms/hands (known as paraesthesia).

The Safe Way

Really the only way to avoid doing this very bad habit is *not* to nod off! *But* if you know that you do have this habit then at least protect your body/neck and ensure you have a neck pillow to prevent the head from dropping forward or drooping to the side. The more mature people should ensure they go to bed after lunch regardless of whether they think they are tired or not, as in my experience, it will soon become clear if they are tired or not when they find themselves waking from that 'forty winks'. As for people in a train/plane/car as a passenger, that's such a difficult one… all I can tell you is the problem it will cause if you do this detrimental habit. I really don't have a magical answer, my advice, just try to keep yourself stimulated enough to stay awake, knowing the consequences should be enough!

45. Pregnancy/beer belly/overweight

Look at any heavily pregnant women who when they stand up will undoubtedly put both hands on either side of the small of their backs to assist them as they straighten themselves up. This is because the person has gained a lot of weight in such a small amount of time and the body is not used to handling such a strain on the low back. The mere fact that she has put her hands on the base of her back indicates where the load is… and this is only usually for the last four out of the nine months!! However, people who are overweight or who have a beer belly are putting a constant strain on the lower back.

The trouble is this kind of weight gain is slow and usually over a prolonged period of time so the person will accommodate the gain, unaware of the pressure they will be putting on the spine (not to mention their joints!). Over time, this strain has a crushing effect on the lower lumbar spinal discs and it is the discs that if they get squashed out of shape protrude into spaces they are not meant to be… these spaces are usually occupied by nerves, which can have dire consequences.

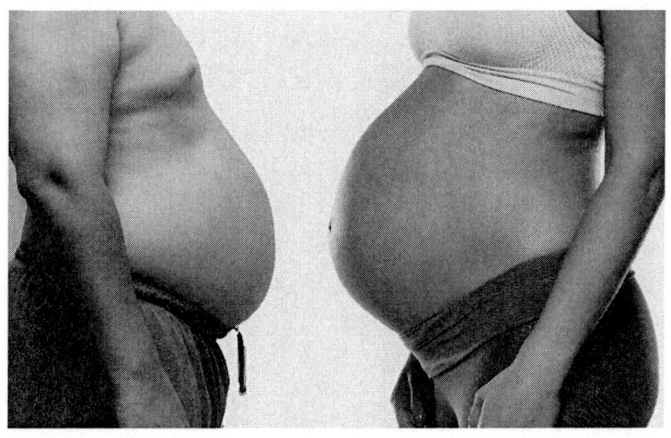

46. Post-natal – carrying your baby

Unfortunately, having a child doesn't come with an instruction manual, so many sleepless nights, being tired and having to manage a completely new way of life gives you an opportunity to create your own shortcuts and bad habits very quickly. So if you are reading this and thinking of having a child, please become wise about the harm shortcuts can cause.

Remember – if it's quicker and easier to do an action – it's usually wrong!
It's not what action you do, it's how you do it.

Carrying a new-born baby is not really a great problem since most babies are a manageable weight and size. However, this condition soon changes and as they quickly grow both in size and weight they begin to wriggle making handling them more challenging. In addition, their attention-seeking capabilities spring into action demanding on an almost seemingly never-ending call of duty! This demand for attention means that the parent has to have one eye on the baby and one doing what they need to e.g., housework, cooking, preparation of baby's milk/meals, etc., so already multitasking has arrived. However, by getting yourself into these good habits before baby comes along then you will be doing them correctly even if you are having to multitask at speed☺. Let us look at some of the new tasks having a baby will present for you.

b. Carrying baby.

Probably the *worst* offender particularly for women since they tend to be the main carers though this trend is now changing, see picture below, where mum has perched the child firmly on her hips. This postural position pushes out the lower spine and with an extra load, in this example of about 14–15 kgs, that's a heck of weight to be throwing the spine out of kilter. If it were just for a one-off, it might not be so bad however, in my own experience and yes, I too was a great offender, this habit is a regular one. Mainly because the woman has a handbag or is carrying something else so finds it easier to plonk the child on a hip… I only wish I knew then what I know now… oh those immortal words!

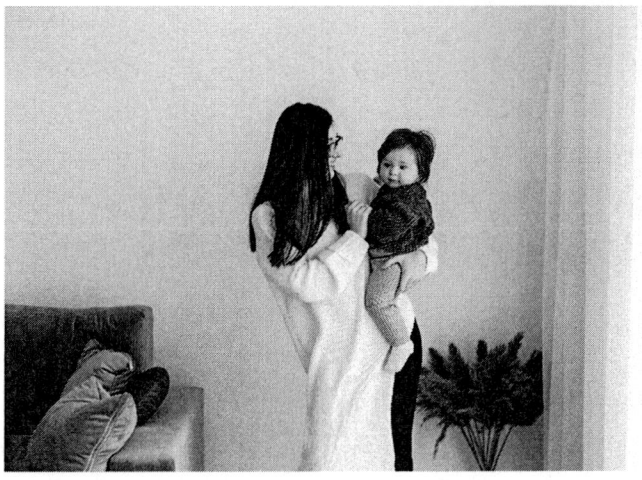

The Safe Way

Carry the child in front of you with both hands. Whilst I know this means both hands are tied, it does mean you are supporting the child correctly with no risk of dropping them and more importantly, no risk to yourself!

b) **Multi-tasking with child.**

The problem here occurs when the person in charge of the household/child tries to do more than one thing at a time. You can see how this is an accident waiting to happen to the child let alone to you! Don't do it. OK, so the child cries, or grizzles, but no one ever got harmed from that, so pop the child in a bouncer maybe in front of a TV or washing machine, as I recall they have a mesmerising effect; then you can perform that task safely.

47. Carrying your child in a car seat

This is a serious problem as you will always have the safety of your baby uppermost in your mind and the safety of you last! But you can and must protect yourself for the sake of your baby. Practice doing the safe actions before your baby arrives so that it will be automatic by the time your baby arrives. Most people will pick up the baby car seat with one hand putting enormous strain on that side of the spine, an accident waiting to happen I'm afraid.

The Safe Way

Is to stand either directly behind or directly in front of the car seat so that the baby can see what you are about to do, bend both your knees whilst keeping your back straight, allow the legs to slowly lower the upper body, secure both hands around the middle part of the handle then using only the legs (quads) to push the upper body back up to standing all the while maintaining a straight back. It might look/feel awkward but it will protect you. Remember practice makes perfect.

48. Putting a baby/child in a car seat.

Firstly, if the child can stand and has started to climb don't be tempted to think you have to lift them into the seat, if they can climb at home they can climb into their seat – though they may need to be enticed into doing so. However, if the child is too young or it is a baby ensure the chair is in situ *before* the child is put in. Go to the side you intend to put the child in, open the door wide and hold the child securely whilst and with the pelvis in neutral, place one foot inside the car and bend the knee of that leg, keep the other foot outside the car so the weight is evenly distributed between feet. Gently put the child in the seat then get into the car with both feet so as to minimise the 'twisting of your back' time while you secure the child instead of getting into the car you can bop down to secure the child. To get the child out simply reverse the process, yes this takes a little longer but remember how many times you would do this activity in a day, week, month, year(s) so believe me it *will* be worth it.

49. Picking a child up from the floor

Most people will just lean over put their hands under the child's armpits and lift. This is so dangerous! This action of loading whilst lifting puts enormous strain on the lower spine and again is an accident waiting to happen. The only saving grace is that people usually have children while they are young, fit and healthy so hopefully, not too much previous damage to the spine has occurred, but this doesn't give you 'carte blanch' to continue doing this bad habit. But beware grandparents!

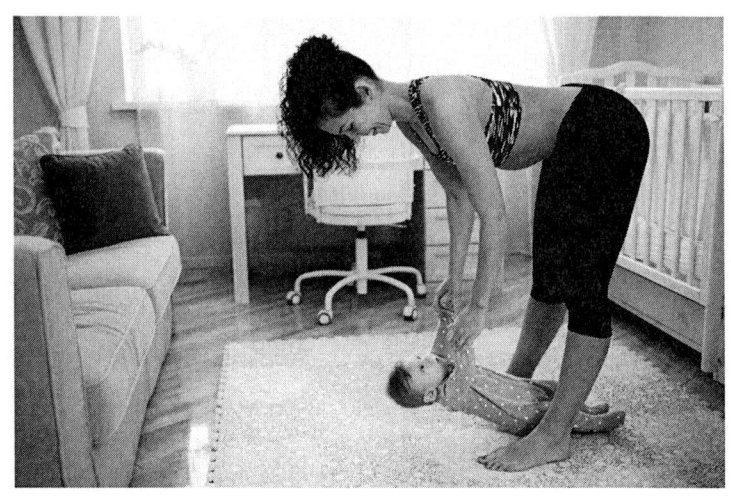

The Safe Way

Is to pick up the child as for the picture below. Alas the majority of parents bend their backs/use their arms to pick up their child – see page 75. Enjoy your child safely!

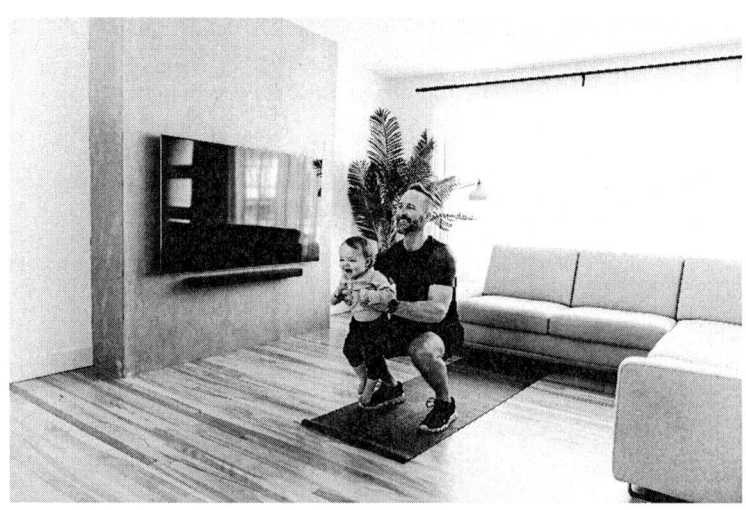

And **men, NEVER** carry a small child on your shoulders! Since your head is forced forward, all the weight of the child is on your neck spine (cervical vertebrae) – we were never intended to carry weight on our necks.

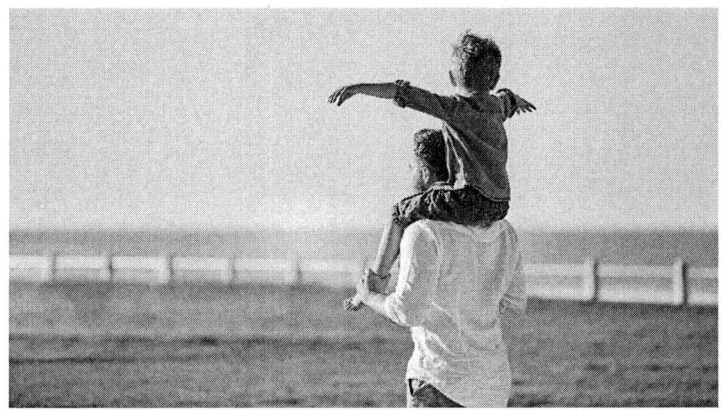

50. Things in the back of the car

If you are in the habit of putting things in the back seat for example your handbag, your laptop, your briefcase, lunch box, etc., that habit is fine as long as you do it correctly. However, if you are sitting in the front seats and merely reach behind you to either get or put the item on the back seat that is putting too much stress load on the upper spine added with the twist needed to do the action it.

The Safe Way

It might seem obvious but the safest way is to open the back door of the car and put your item(s) on the back seat and reverse the process when you get to your destination. This does not involve any twisting at all.

My tip: Remember if you put things on the back seat they can be seen and accessible when you stop at traffic lights/junctions – beware opportunists! Best keep valuables in the boot.

51. Driving a car – 1

It may sound silly to have to mention this but you would be very surprised how many people do this particular bad habit, especially if you own an automatic. When on a long journey when top gear has been reached the right foot is engaged on the accelerator, however, the left leg 'rests' in the foot well, trouble is it leans against it at an outward angle (we call that externally rotated) this puts immediate pressure on the very last two vertebrae in your back (the ones that are known to cause the majority of all back problems!)

The Safe Way

The easiest way to get out of this habit is to bend the knee so the foot is flat on the floor, ensuring the seat is in the upright position will help maintain the correct posture. It takes the strain off the low back you will be doing yourself a huge favour especially if your job/hobby involves driving on a regular basis.

52. Driving a car – 2

If you are the sort of person who drives with the window down and rests the elbow on the door frame then – stops it immediately. What you are doing is repetitively lifting only the right elbow to fit onto the door, this raises the right shoulder (steering wheel on the right). OK for a one-off but in my experience it is more of a habit for people who regularly drive a car e.g. a taxi driver, delivery 'white van man', etc. because the shoulder is raised it shortens the upper back muscle fibres on that side creating an imbalance with the other side stressing the load carried at the neck and shoulder/arm.

The Safe Way

If you don't do this then please don't be tempted to start this habit, it will create problems in the long term, besides both hands should be firmly fixed on the steering wheel anyway!

Remember – if it's quicker and easier to do an action – it's usually wrong!
It's not what action you do, it's how you do it.

53. Driving a car – 3

And speaking of hands on the wheel. So many of the men I have seen drive with their arms straight and locked at the elbow with their car seats tilted right back at an obtuse angle of about 130 degrees! It might look cool but boy is it taking its toll on your back both straining between the shoulder blades and the low back, so congratulations you are managing to muck up all your spine up in one go!

The Safe Way

Try to get your seat as upright as possible and realise that nowadays most cars steering wheel adjusts so when you are seated comfortably you can adjust your steering wheel up/down and in/out to suit you so your arms are bent at the elbow. The crown of your head should rest against the head restraint while driving, this will keep it in the neutral position and stop it from wandering forward.

My Tip – Don't be tempted to leave your left hand on the gear stick, this puts onus on the right hand to grip the steering wheel.

54. <u>Driving a car – 4. Reversing</u>

If you are in the habit of sitting in the driver's seat, then either twisting your head or worse twisting your body while putting the left arm on the passenger seat and using only the right hand to do the manoeuvre you will have strained the lower back considerably.

The Safe Way

When reversing try to use the mirrors that way your head will be facing forwards and you will only be using your eyes.

55. <u>Car – Shopping</u>

If like me, you tend to overload your shopping bags in the hope that you won't have to carry too many. It never works out that way, does it? We all buy more than we need. We then gather up the bags and dump them in the car boot. When we get home we try to carry as much as we can at one hit in an attempt to save return trips to the car. Sound familiar? Well to be honest if you have anything other than an estate car, where you can drag the shopping to the edge and then lift, you will be lifting your shopping in/out of the car with jerky type movements which use mainly your lower back, since you are leaning over and your spine will be out of ninety (see next chapter)

The Safe Way

Don't be tempted to overload the bags in the first instance. Secondly, treat the expedition as exercise so the more times you go to the car the more calories you burn up. Lastly, in order to lift correctly, you will need to put your pelvis in neutral to prevent your lower back from coming into play when you lift at this angle. Once your pelvis is in neutral you can then pull the shopping as close to the opening of the boot as you can and then lift with your arms. As they won't be as heavy you will be able to avoid the jerking movement. When putting the bags down, use the bended knees movement to lower your upper body with the bags to the floor.

56. Leaning – 1

It is a well-known fact that middle-aged men, in particular, would fall over if they didn't have anything to lean on/against. Why they have to do this is beyond me but do it they do; using one hand to lean up against they usually cross one foot over the other ankle so the whole spine is curved. It could be a signpost, a wall, a door jamb, a counter, a shovel, a broom, in fact anything and if these aren't available then it's another person (usually the little woman). They do not seem to be able to stand on both feet. Ladies just be aware of your men and tell me if I'm not right!

The Safe Way

Is not to lean obviously, however, easier said than done if it has been your lifetime's habit! Try to stand with your feet wider apart than usual this will help prevent you over leaning and get your partners to point out when you are doing it.

57. Leaning – 2

The other type of leaning we all do is with our waists up against a sink/worktop when doing actions like washing up, preparing vegetables, at a workbench. Most of us are unaware we actually do this but I think you will find we all do… yes even me! When we lean onto our hip bones we put pressure onto the lower spine. Regularly done this will put a strain on that part of the body.

The Safe Way

Stand slightly away from the sink and bend the knees slightly to 'soften' them. This ensures your back will remain straight and you won't be leaning on the surface.

58. Getting in/out of the bath

Most people just step over the side of the bath and then lower themselves into the bath using their hands on the sides of the bath. And then reverse this process to get up/out of the bath.

This puts excess strain on the arms (shoulders in particular) and is very dangerous since the majority of us use bubble baths or soap that creates an ice-rink effect on the bath base. In addition, the reason most of us push up on our shoulders is that the large muscles in the legs (quads) aren't strong enough to push our bodyweight upwards!

The Safe Way

Build up those quads! (See the section on exercises)

To get in the bath hold onto the sides and step into the bath keeping hold of the sides, lower your body, so you go onto your knees and then sit in the bath. NB if you are a mature citizen, you would do well to have a bath anti-slip mat on the bath floor.

To get out of the bath, drain All the bathwater before attempting to get up. Then sit up and use your hands to steady you on the sides of the bath or handrails, turn yourself over onto your knees and using the large quad muscles push your body upwards only using your hands to steady yourself.

59. Wearing glasses

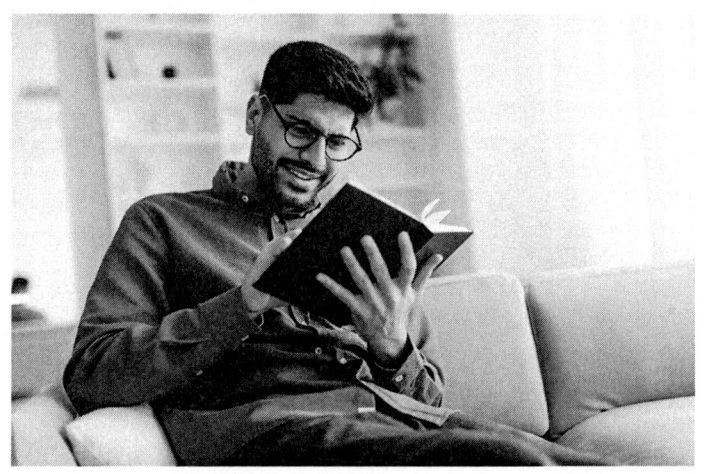

If you wear multi-focal lenses, you should have been taught to move your head to view, rather than your eyes, since the latter will cause your eyes to look through the prism and this has the same effect as being on a merry-go-round and can cause nausea and headaches. However, moving your head may entice you to look down at your work (refer to bad habits number 14). For wearers of ordinary or bifocal glasses, when you need to read you tend to tip your head to be able to look through your glasses, this definitely bends the head. If you do this regularly, you will be creating a bad habit (picture above)

The Safe Way

By putting your glasses on the end of your nose and keeping your head up and back you can use your eyes to look down through the glasses to read the item if it can't be raised to eye height. However, the majority of times it is easier to take the item to your eyes simply lift the book, phone, iPad, newspaper, etc., to your eyes. You can use a cushion on your lap or as I do, when sitting, hold the book in your hands and secure the elbows into the waste which acts as a book rest and as the pillow, is quite comfortable for long periods of time. Whatever method you choose, ensure the item is eye height.

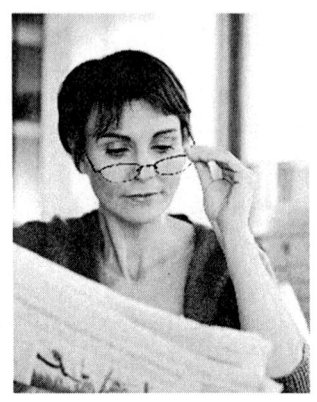

60. Taking jumpers/shirts on/off

Most people put a jumper on by pushing the head through the top and then feeding individual arms into the sleeves. But when it comes to taking it off the arms cross over in front of you and grabbing opposite sides of the jumper and then pulling it upwards over the head. This puts enormous strain on the shoulder joints.

The Safe Way

Simply reverse how you put it on. That is, take each arm out of the sleeve, and then lift the neck of the jumper over the head (most women who have 'hair-do's' will automatically take them off this way).

And finally… Getting on/off a chair

I have covered a fair few bad habits so far and it is my hope that by now you will be able to apply the new habits learned to other similar actions to protect your body/spine from now on. However, I have *left this bad habit to the last for good reason*. In my experience, this bad habit causes more serious damage to the body than ***any*** other I have come across, especially since the majority of older people have sadly resorted to this. It is the years of bending the back over rather than bopping down when we do an action, that has weakened/atrophied the most important muscles in the body, the Quadriceps muscles (quads), located in the front upper thighs. These muscles are the ones that *would have* supported your body when you need them most, for example, if you start to fall. The quads engage strongly when you brace yourself using your foot, this would normally stop the body's forward momentum and prevent your fall!!! However, because the leg muscles are so weak they don't work in this way and so can't stop you from falling, what happens is the momentum propels you forward until you crash into something and stop or fall on the floor.

Getting up from a chair

If you have ever watched your elderly parents/grandparents getting on/off chairs, you will have noticed that they put both hands firmly on the arm rest of the chair or their laps and push hard on their arms in order to lift their upper bodies out of the chair. Now since their arms are only so long, they can't push themselves up to vertical, and so at this point, they are now stuck halfway up and halfway down. In order to continue upwards they then launch themselves forward out of the chair and attempt to walk straight away, the quads are not strong enough to push them up so the person, already in motion continues taking numerous tiny steps in a forward momentum while at the same time trying to gradually straighten up their upper bodies until finally, they are standing up.

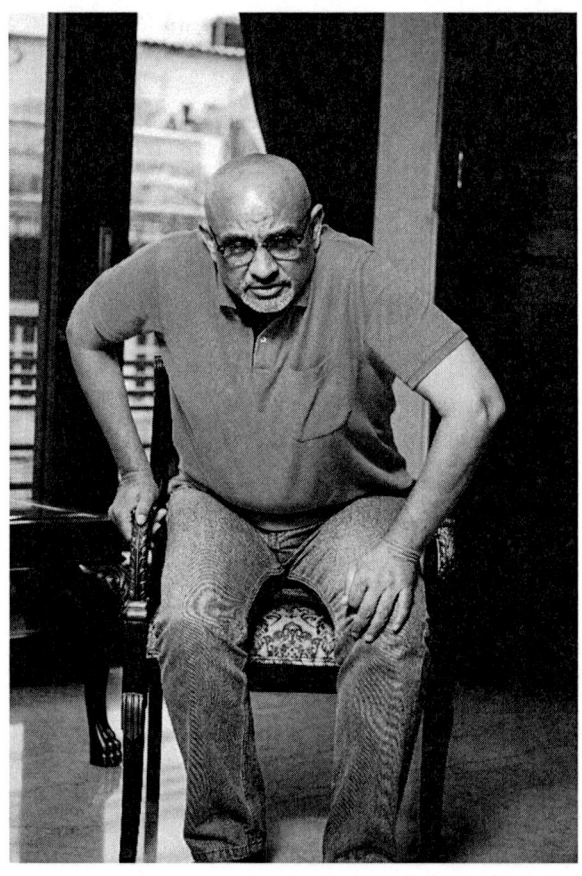

Because they are still moving forward only luck or an object will allow them to stop! All because they have *lost* the power in their quads and have no strength in them to push their upper body weight out of the chair.

Sitting in the chair is far easier for the elderly since they hold onto the chair armrests, ensuring the back of their legs are touching the seat of the chair, they then allow gravity to lower their upper bodies onto the seat, usually with a hard uncontrolled plonk! Not exactly elegant but I guess the objective has been achieved.

The Safe Way

The elderly will need to build up those quads before they can attempt this, but if they still have use of their thigh muscles then please get them to change this habit NOW…

Ensure you are not using your hands at all (I advise to clasp them together in front of you this prevents you from being tempted to use them), gently lean forward, then use a slight rocking motion, whilst at the same time pushing *straight up* with your upper thighs (quads). Do Not be tempted to move off the spot or walk *until* your upper body is fully vertical! Once it is, only then should you start to walk as you will now be fully in control of your body. Just keep doing it you will get there in the end.

57b Sitting down

I guess most of you will probably reach for the arms of the chair to ensure that you can feel the back of the chair on your legs before you sit down, then allow gravity to seat you i.e., you sit down with a 'plonk'. Well, you are halfway there to a new habit… However, when your knees are touching the back of the chair, in this position clasp your hands in front of you (so you are not tempted to reach for the arms of the chair) then with control, slowly lower your upper body onto the seat. You will 'plonk' down at first, however, using this new habit will strengthen those weak quads and in time you will have full control to sit down on (and get up off) the chair properly.

Remember: Practice Makes Perfect and Prevents Injury!

Review of the Chapter

- **It's not *what* action you do – it's *how* you do it.**
- **An action that is quicker and easier to do is usually wrong.**
- When doing an action *think* about how to do it safely.
- Don't try to correct all your bad habits at once – you will overload yourself and ultimately fail!
- Only change your top *three* habits at a time (from your priority list) in order to guarantee your success.
- Praise yourself when you get things right.
- Changing any of your habits will feel strange at first but by using the 'how to change a habit' and 'Carrie's rule of ninety' in chapter seven you will get there in the end.
- Practice makes perfect and will prevent injury.

Chapter 7
How to Change Your Habits and Carrie's 'Rule of Ninety'

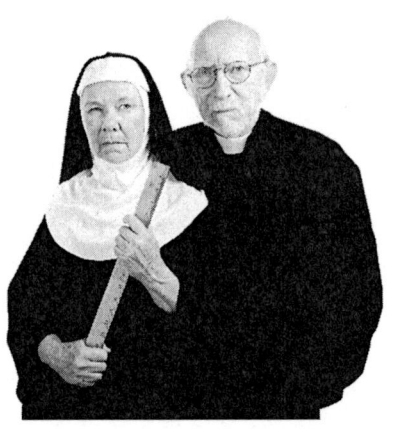

As we now know habits are actions that are repetitive; that when first done, if they produce no threat to our body, that is, produce no disastrous consequences of that action, the brain deems that action as being 'safe' to perform and so allows us to repeat the action again and again. I hope by now having identified your own bad habits, you are much wiser to the fact that this is definitely not the case!

In order to change a bad habit, we need to know the correct way of doing that action, repeat it and allow it to become our new habit. A lot of these habits were identified in the previous chapter. Most of the time we can change the bad habits gradually as told in the previous chapter by picking ourselves up and repeating that action at least 1000 times or regularly for a short period of time. But this is all well and good knowing how to correct the faults when you are awake but how do you do so for bad habits when you are asleep?

How To Change a Habit

(Conscious or Subconscious)

When an action is performed repetitively with no dire consequences, the body deems that action as safe and allows us to repeat it. The brain allows us to store that information in the subconscious so that we perform that action repeatedly and it becomes 'automatic' for example, we don't have to tell our legs to walk because we have learned this action after repeatedly falling, stumbling when we were very young now we do it 'without thinking about it' (automatically). However, it *doesn't* make the action we learned right!

You may be aware that people can learn new things while they are asleep by playing audible tapes to themselves throughout the night, this is because the subconscious is continually working on our behalf. So in order to *change a habit,* we need to talk to the subconscious. The technique to do this is below, just follow the instructions implicitly... trust me... it really works; I know I have done it and changed several of mine!

The technique to use to change a habit

In order to *change* a bad habit, you will need to *demonstrate* to the body what that habit is. Look at yourself in a mirror demonstrating the bad habit and say out loud to your mirrored self, "It is dangerous for my body to do this action."

Repeat the action this time saying, "The body must stop me from doing this action in the future as it is harmful for it."

Now demonstrate the *correct* action at the same time say to yourself in the mirror, "It is safe for my body to do *this* action."

Repeat the good action whilst saying, "This action must be done in the future to keep my body safe."

Carrie's Rule of Ninety

We can see that the human body stands upright in line with gravity and the angle created is ninety degrees with the ground i.e. we are perpendicular with gravity. The skeleton and musculature of the body have been designed/formulated throughout time to hold us in that straight upward position ensuring that the loading on the joints is equalled throughout the body.

I have studied loading on the human body and found that if we keep the body as close to multiples of ninety degrees as possible, the loading is distributed safely. Let me explain (see diagram on next page). We shall start from the base. When seated we need to keep the feet pointing directly forward, this means they are at ninety degrees to the shin bones. It is important to have the correct height chair, that is, one that allows the knee bend to be at ninety degrees to the hip bone, the back is then straight upwards at ninety degrees to the thigh bone. The head stays tall while the chin is pulled back so is in a neutral position. This keeps the head equalled so its loading is half over your front and half over your back. Your shoulders will need to be kept in neutral that is, not allowed to roll forward (round-shouldered) thus completing the seated rule of ninety.

Standing rule of ninety

Again, the feet are pointing straight forward at ninety degrees to the ankle bone, feet should be hip width apart allowing the body's weight to be evenly distributed between both feet. The hips should be in pelvic neutral (you should feel slight tension in your abdomen and in your upper thighs and buttocks), your back is straight upward, shoulders straight and head in neutral (see the picture in chapter 2 – 'good posture') My tip – When your head is in neutral it is anatomically impossible to let the shoulders round (come forwards)... try it and see... However, if you let the head go forward the shoulders will also be allowed to round, this puts unnecessary pressure at the base of the neck between the upper part of the shoulder blades. Repeating this bad habit will create pressure on the cervical/brachial plexus that feeds the neck, shoulders, arms and hands so any of these can be affected when the nerve pathway is irritated. So watch that head.

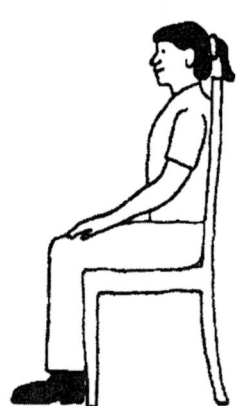

Exercises

As already identified, the majority of problems occur from wrongful bending of our backs, this weakens the quadriceps muscles which are needed to push up your upper body. In order that you may employ good habits, you will first need to strengthen these muscles. It is a simple exercise to do but must be done regularly.

Quadriceps exercise Stand with your heels against the skirting board, feet hip width apart and keeping your head, shoulders and upper body against the wall (but NOT leaning on the wall), keeping your heels on the floor at all times slowly lower your upper body by bending your knees.

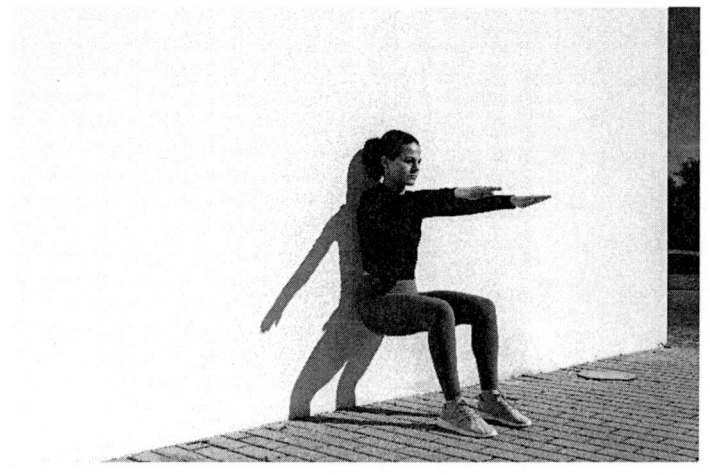

Keep your back against the wall at all times, Slide down as far as you can. Use your front thighs to push yourself back up.

Don't go down too far (at first, since it makes the next part harder to do), now push yourself up to the starting position again. Repeat this 10 times, have a rest and then do another 10, rest and finally another set of 10 that is, 30 in total. This will take only a few minutes and can be done against any wall or a securely closed door. If you do this twice a day, you will eventually get further and further down the wall as your quads get stronger and stronger then sitting and standing will become easier and easier.

The Stomach is also important in supporting the spine since muscles work in pairs. The tighter the abdominals the better protection for the spine. This is a very simple exercise for anyone to do of any age!

Stomach exercises – 1

Lie on the floor with knees bent, feet flat on the floor and hip width apart. With straight arms put the hands on your thighs palm side down. Take a breath in and on the out breath, slide the hands up the thighs making sure your chin is tucked into your chest as your head and shoulders come off the floor. Breathe in and slowly roll back down to the starting position. Try to do 10 x three times.

The aim is to do this exercise in a controlled manner and to get up and over the knee, hold the position at the knee for a count of 5 then slowly with control, slide back down.

Once the above is achieved you can increase the repetitions in sets of 5 or 10. This exercise protects the spine. If you have rounded shoulders, you might need a pillow under your head as support.

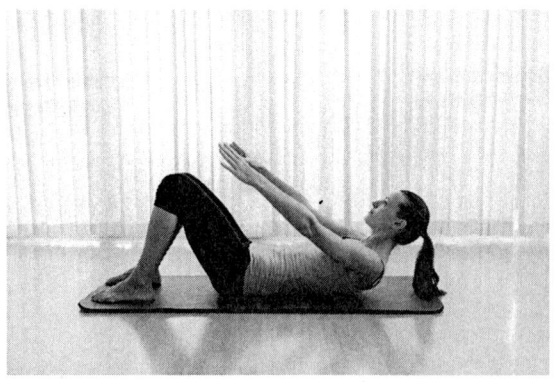

Stomach exercise – 2

The plank – Whilst there are various forms of doing the plank, I will teach the basic form which will be sufficient to maintain a healthy body. Lie on your front arms shoulder-width apart with elbows bent and palms of hands flat on the floor. Legs stretched out behind you, turn your toes down to the ground, now in this position tighten your tummy and buttocks and lift your whole body off the floor. Keep the head facing the floor and the spine in alignment – hold this position until you get a shake in your tummy, bend the knees to rest. Do NOT hold your breath when doing this exercise, just breathe normally. At first, you may only be able to obtain the starting position, but as you practice you will be able to stay in the plank position longer and longer until you build up to a minute. This is all the time you need to maintain good health.

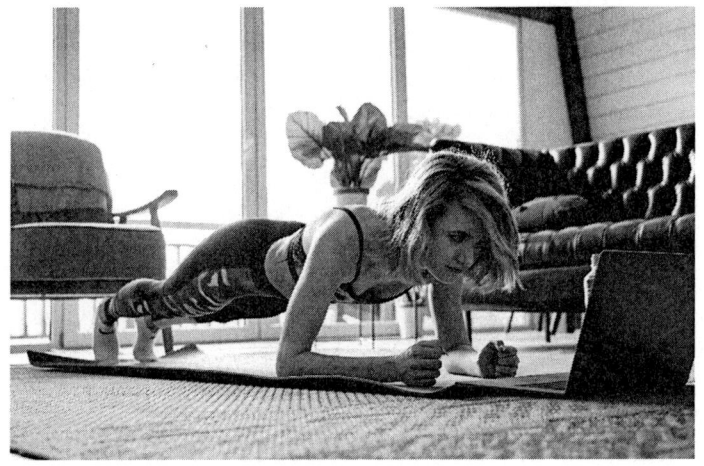

Remember!
If it's quicker and easier to do an action – it's usually wrong!
It's not what action you do, it's how you do it.

Review of the Chapter

- Habits are learned responses. Therefore, if we accept this, then we must accept that they can be <u>Un</u> learned.
- To change a habit, it takes 1000 repetitions or 2-8 months
- Don't get frustrated if things don't go as fast as you want them to, simply reflect on how long it has taken you to get where you are now (all your life!) and give yourself a pat on the back for your efforts!
- Replace your bad habits with good ones.
- Remember you must tell your subconscious out loud what it NEEDS to do! It won't let you down!
- Apply Carrie's rule of ninety for the majority of your actions and you will achieve much.
- Exercise those quads and Abs three times daily… these powerful exercises will change your life!

Chapter 8
Other Factors Affecting Posture

During my many years as a specialist in musculoskeletal problems I discovered that the majority of problems caused by bad posture come from these sources:

1. The person will have developed bad posture from 'quick fixes' and 'short cuts' doing an action for themselves.
2. Learned the bad habit from being taught or observing an action that a peer is doing.
3. A structural problem (skeletal) caused initial pain or discomfort and this made the body/person alter their posture to get away from the pain or discomfort (known as postural compensation).

It is unfortunate that the UK NHS do not readily accept that the spine and its compartments; vertebrae, discs and nerves, can (and in my experience do), cause many problems and pain in the human body. For example: Lumbar vertebra 5 (known as L5) if rotated out of its normal position (known as a misalignment), inflames the corresponding disc which can press on its nerve pathway creating pain *anywhere* along that pathway depending on how much of the nerve is pinched/affected by the rotation. The pain pathway of L5 can affect the buttock, the inside of the knee, the outside of the calf (often manifesting itself as a cramp-like pain), irritation and or pain across the top of the ankle (resemble a tight band feeling) and pain or discomfort under the ball of the foot (often misdiagnosed as plantar fasciitis). There may not be any pain in your back, in addition, the body may have already compensated for the misalignment and laid down a protective fibrous coating around the vertebra. This masks and often eases the symptoms.

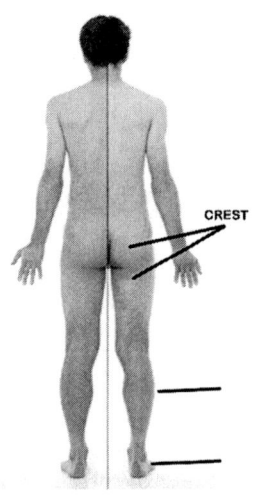

L5 nerve pathway:

The bony part of iliac and under buttock

outer part of calf

ball of foot and big toe

Should you suspect there may be a problem with your back OR your symptoms are not getting any better despite medical intervention it is well worth getting a consultation with a recommended person such as an Osteopath who will be able to assess you better. Unfortunately, it is rare (in my experience) for any NHS spinal 'specialist' to even know, let alone accept that vertebrae can rotate out of their position, therefore the chances of them knowing about the symptoms and pain they cause or their pain pathways are slim to nil, let alone know how to correct the problem!

Regrettably, I have wasted many hours writing letters to NHS Doctors and consultants informing them that patients of 'ours' whom they have told to 'learn to live with their pain', have been successfully treated at my clinic because an accurate diagnosis has been made to find the cause of their pain and its origin! This surely highlights the need to look at what the NHS professionals are being taught at grass roots in medical school?

Vertebral rotations create disc bulging that cause nerve innervation which in turn causes muscle spasms and pain, the body reacts to pain by moving away from it so it doesn't hurt anymore. This is known as postural compensation. It is this postural compensation that creates an imbalance of muscles and joint loading, that in time will cause other problems and so we compensate again and thus create a cycle of causing pain and moving away from it. This is why the accurate initial diagnosis of the cause of a presenting problem is imperative to stop this cycle and prevent further injuries occurring: -

Repetitive bad habit (action) → trauma of some kind = last straw → rotation of spine → pain → pain killers → formation of scar tissue for protection → postural compensation while scar tissue forms → no pain → compensated action continues → imbalance → new problem starting...

I have known patients present with a problem they have had for years, yet during the intensive consultation, I discover they have a multitude of problems, mainly compensatory! Although these will have been a contributory factor to their current presenting problem, in order to sort out their present problem, I have to correct *all* of them! Thankfully we are living tissue, so with time, correct treatment and much prayer it is possible to reverse the damage done, improving the range of movements, posture but most importantly alleviating their pain while improving their quality of life.

Occupations can influence our posture, for example, electricians, plumbers, carpet layers to name just a few, who put their bodies into the most precarious positions demonstrating nearly all the bad habits at once! However, some jobs demand that position and unfortunately, there is no way out. These types of vocations highlight how essential it is for these tradespeople to maintain good postural positions when they are *not* at work!

Final Thoughts

In our daily lives, the actions we do mean that we use certain muscles more than others. The ones we don't use become weak so it is important to be aware of the ones we don't use and strengthen them. However, we have identified it is the quadriceps muscles that will provide the best protection for your body as they are used to enable you to squat, rise from sitting, save you when you stumble, push up when you kneel down, get in and out of a bath, etc. These muscles will save your spine from overuse and damage! So just keep practising the new habits, don't forget the golden rules below but most of all, pass on the knowledge you now have learned to loved ones and friends so they don't end up with future problems.

Remember:

If it's quicker and easier to do an action – it's usually wrong!
It's not what action you do, it's how you do it.

Bibliography

Lally. Phillipa. HuffPost, healthy living, Oct 27, 2014. Health psychology researcher at University College London. A study published in the *European Journal of Social Psychology*.

Sissons Claire – (online article) MedialNewsToday, Feb 7, 2020 What are refined carbohydrates.

Other books by Carrie Ransom

The Sepia Technique – A technique I developed that Clears the lymph Nodes, unlike the conventional manual lymphatic Drainage, performed only on the limbs. My technique restores the immune system, reverses poor health, detoxes your body and improves your quality of life.